A MOST QUIET MURDER

A MOST QUIET MURDER

MATERNITY, AFFLICTION, AND VIOLENCE IN LATE NINETEENTH-CENTURY FRANCE

SUSANNAH WILSON

CORNELL UNIVERSITY PRESS
Ithaca and London

First published 2025 by Cornell University Press

Library of Congress Cataloging-in-Publication Data

Names: Wilson, Susannah, 1976– author.
Title: A most quiet murder : maternity, affliction, and
    violence in late nineteenth-century France / Susannah
    Wilson.
Description: Ithaca : Cornell University Press, 2025. |
    Includes bibliographical references and index.
Identifiers: LCCN 2025003330 (print) | LCCN 2025003331
    (ebook) | ISBN 9781501784224 (hardcover) | ISBN
    9781501784231 (epub) | ISBN 9781501784248 (pdf)
Subjects: LCSH: Murder—France—Dijon—History—19th
    century—Case studies | Women—France—Social
    conditions—19th century. | Poor women—France—
    Social conditions—19th century. | LCGFT: Case studies.
Classification: LCC HV6535.F8 D595 2025 (print) | LCC
    HV6535.F8 (ebook)
LC record available at https://lccn.loc.gov/2025003330
LC ebook record available at https://lccn.loc.gov/2025003331

For David

Contents

PREFACE

In the early months of 2024, as I was putting the finishing touches to this manuscript, my husband found an old handbag in the attic of his parents' house. It had once belonged to his grandmother Alice. My father-in-law was born in 1939, the youngest by ten years of a long line of siblings (perhaps eight or nine, nobody can ever remember). The handbag contained old letters, postcards, black-and-white photographs, and other miscellaneous papers. Among these were some commemorative cards recording the births, names, and deaths of three of the five children Alice had lost. Although infant mortality rates were much higher in the early twentieth century, it was still unusual for a woman to lose five children—to prematurity, disease, and accidents. My father-in-law has no recollection of his mother talking about these siblings who died before he was born, and he does not remember their names. This tall, sturdy, handsome woman from the East End of London (the most populous working-class district of any city in Europe at the time) just carried on and looked to the future, caring for the family she had, uncomplaining, grateful that her other children had survived. But she kept those little slips of paper until she died in 1990, at the age of ninety, which suggests that she always quietly remembered the ones who had not lived long. Still, we know nothing of how she bore the pain of her losses—for painful it must have been. Her story mirrors the experiences of so many women from the near past who gave birth to numerous children, many of whom had remarkably short lives.

Each woman's pregnancy involves a full nine months of physical and emotional investment as well as a certain level of risk; if the birth goes ahead without major complications, in normal circumstances the result is an intense attachment between mother and child. At least, this is what is culturally expected of mothers. The loss of a child is, therefore, a profound emotional wrench. Psychologists sometimes conceive of it in terms of trauma. Some women are temperamentally resilient, process the shock quickly, and remain optimistic about life and the future. Others, perhaps highly sensitive, remember the experience as though it were yesterday and continue to feel intense sadness even years later. A small number of women respond to the loss of a child in ways that are culturally taboo. This book tells the dramatic and intriguing story of a woman who, it seems, reacted to the death of an infant in an extraordinary way—not with sorrow, heartbreak, love, or resilience but with violence and, at times, callous indifference.

As with so many microhistorical investigations—designed to draw out the particularities of a single case and moment of crisis, to illuminate a wider historical moment—the story told here was inspired by an accidental find. I was working on another as-yet unfinished book on the cultural history of morphine in late nineteenth-century France, and in my reading of the contemporary medical literature on opiates I chanced upon an unusual story. The medical doctor and scholar Henri Guimbail, who specialized in drug and alcohol detoxification treatments, included a brief reference to the "Fiquet affair" in his 1891 paper, "Crimes et délits commis par les morphinomanes," published in the prominent medical journal the *Annales d'hygiène publique et de médecine légale*. This citation piqued my interest in the reverberations of a now-forgotten case, which had briefly opened up to public examination the intimate lives of people whose existence would otherwise have passed into obscurity. The case concerned a woman named Marie-Françoise Fiquet who was accused of abducting and killing a five-year-old girl in the French city of Dijon in the summer of 1882. Her actions seemed cruel, gratuitous, and motiveless, and the initial focus of the investigation was on the suspect's drug addiction and its possibly deranging effects. However, from an initial reading of the material, it seemed to me that this was a red herring, that her crime and her morphine addiction were both distantly connected to her own experience of child loss and to the everyday physical pains and economic struggles of working women's lives. In pursuit of this hypothesis, I located the original *dossier de procédure* in the Archives Départementales de la Côte-d'Or in Dijon. Its fragile and crumbling papers had been placed into a stiff cardboard file that I suspect had remained closed since Fiquet's conviction in 1883. The file contained the interrogations, witness statements, letters, autopsy reports, and other miscellaneous evidence used to build the case against the accused woman and her husband. The archivists in Dijon were immensely helpful with my search, as were the librarians at the Bibliothèque nationale de France, without whom I would have had great difficulty locating the regional press reports and the goldmine of information contained in Émile Mermet's independently published multivolume work, the *Annuaire de la presse française* (1883).

This project has been a work in progress for several years, and I have shared my ideas informally with colleagues and formally with sympathetic audiences at conferences and seminars held by academic societies in the United Kingdom and the United States: Nineteenth-Century French Studies, the Society for the Study of French History, and the Alcohol and Drugs History Society. This research and my broader network organization and research on drugs in nineteenth-century France has also been made possible by funding awards from the British Academy, the Leverhulme Trust, and my home institution, the University of Warwick, which has also supported me with generous periods of institutional leave. I have benefited enormously from intellectual engagement with friends and colleagues in French Studies, Gender Studies, Anthropology, and French History who have discussed my ideas with me, offered hospitality in France, or read early drafts of the material presented in this book. All the feedback they offered was thoughtful, brilliantly incisive, and above all encouraging. In no particular order, thanks are due to Jeremy Ahearne, Sara E. Black, Miranda Gill, Lisa Downing, Christina de Bellaigue, Caroline Warman, Maya Mayblin, Kate Astbury, Oliver Davis, Jessica Wardhaugh, Seán Hand, Pierre-Philippe Fraiture, Nicolas Kasprzyk, Magalie Simeray, Annie Rogge, and Odile Krakovitch. I am also grateful to my editor at Cornell University Press, Bethany Wasik, and the two anonymous readers, for the care and attention they have given to the project. My biggest debt of thanks is owed to my family: my mother, Mavis Wilson, came with me to Dijon to visit the town and the archives, and has taken a lively interest in the story told here; my children, Nathaniel and Genevieve, have grown tall while I have been writing this book and have been a noisy but happy distraction from writing; and finally, my patient husband, David Boyd Haycock, has been an exacting reader and editor and an unwavering support on the home front. The book is dedicated to him, with love and thanks.

NOTE ON THE TEXT
AND SOURCES

This book tells the story of a married couple who were accused of murdering a child, Henriette Barbey, in Dijon in 1882. Their names were Marie-Françoise Rémond, the main suspect, and Pierre Fiquet, her husband and alleged accomplice. In France, in official documents (death certificates, passports, and criminal proceedings) married women are listed under their maiden names. In the documentation relating to the investigation, to indicate married status, the accused woman was referred to as "Marie-Françoise Rémond, femme Fiquet." This was frequently shortened to "la femme Fiquet" or "épouse [spouse/wife] Fiquet." In the sources analyzed here, she is most often called "la femme Fiquet," and the case is known as "L'affaire Fiquet" or "L'affaire des époux Fiquet." Working-class women would not usually have been addressed using the title "Madame," a marker of respect reserved for higher-class women. For this reason, and because the accused woman went by the name of Fiquet (and not Rémond) in everyday life, I refer to her as "Marie-Françoise Fiquet," "the femme Fiquet," or simply "Fiquet." To avoid any ambiguity, I refer to Pierre Fiquet using his full name or Monsieur/Mr. Fiquet. I have also retained the designation "femme" to refer to the other working women who appear in the story (as they were called in the official documentation). In translations of portions of text where the accused woman is named "la femme Fiquet" I have retained the French, italicizing the word *femme* to indicate where this occurs, because there is no equivalent of this naming convention in English, and "Mrs. Fiquet," which sounds polite in English and not procedural, does not quite render it accurately.

The prosecution file, the *dossier de procédure*, is held in the Archives Départementales de la Côte-d'Or in Dijon (abbreviated to ADCO). The file contains two main folders. The first, "Pièces de Procédure," contains the witness statements, interrogations of the suspects, police notes, and other reports such as the autopsy report and the first unpublished psychiatric report by Dr. Émile Blanche. The second, "Renseignements de moralité," contains the collected statements, letters, and allegations specifically about Marie-Françoise Fiquet's character. The spelling of names often varies in archival documentation, especially between the original paperwork and the press reports. I have opted to use the spellings given in original statements and letters, which are signed by all parties and most likely to be accurate.

Dramatis Personae

Family Members, Workers, and Key Witnesses

Marie-Françoise Rémond, femme Fiquet—the accused woman

Pierre Fiquet—husband of Marie-Françoise Fiquet; the co-accused

Marie-Louise Fiquet—daughter of Marie-Françoise Fiquet; legally adopted by Pierre Fiquet

Olympe Tissot, femme Barbey—Henriette's mother

Athanäse Barbey—Henriette's father

Veuve Barbey (widow Barbey)—Henriette's aunt and a neighbor of the Fiquet family

Francine Barreau—Henriette Barbey's five-year-old classmate and witness to her abduction

Louise Coquereaux—fourteen-year-old tobacco-factory worker

Henri Gallimard—ropemaker at the Canal de Bourgogne

Edmé Michel—customs (octroi) officer at the Canal de Bourgogne

Vincent Schettine—silversmith

Marie Fenet—the femme Fiquet's niece

Marie Cagnard—Fiquet family neighbor

Femme Vauthier—Fiquet family neighbor

Femme Lefebvre—Fiquet family neighbor

Dr. Michelot—young medical intern in Dijon

The Abbé Pihéry—Catholic priest in Besançon

Marie-Françoise Fiquet's Alleged Victims

Henriette Barbey—five-year-old girl, found dead in Dijon on 29 June 1882

Mademoiselle Franchinal—young mother of twin babies allegedly "adopted" by the femme Fiquet

Mademoiselle Bautut—young woman; victim of intimate assault and attempted abortion

Mademoiselle Vacherot—young woman; victim of poisoning

Mademoiselle Vallangin—spinster and Spiritist; possible victim of poisoning

Justine and Maria Jobard—teenage sisters and orphanage residents; victims of attempted abduction

Pauline Mugnier—two-year-old girl; victim of attempted abduction

The Investigators

Alfred Loiseau—the *juge d'instruction* (examining magistrate)

Dr. Deroye—local doctor who carried out the autopsy on Henriette Barbey's body

Philippe-Gustave Héberd—chemist and professor at the École de médecine; assisted with the autopsy

Dr. Évariste Marandon de Montyel—psychiatrist (alienist); director of the Chartreuse asylum and examining physician

Dr. Antoine Émile Blanche—psychiatrist (alienist) in Paris; examining physician at Saint-Lazare prison

Étienne Metman—the femme Fiquet's attorney for the defense

Paul Cunisset—Pierre Fiquet's attorney for the defense

M. l'avocat-général Mairet—attorney for the prosecution

Introduction
"The Most Monstrous Crime"

In the early hours of Friday, 30 June 1882, a passing workman discovered the body of a young girl lying on the left bank of the Canal de Bourgogne at the southwestern edge of Dijon, a small city in the east of France. It had been a warm, drizzly evening and the child had been dead for just a few hours. She had apparently drowned, although, curiously, her clothes were still dry.[1] The canal at this location is over twenty yards wide; its breadth and generous, barren banks today lend the area a feeling of emptiness, of urban desolation. Between ten and eleven o'clock that evening, a few people had been milling around: shift workers engaged at their canal-side workshops, such as the fodder suppliers and the candle manufacturers, and young people socializing. Henri Gallimard, a ropemaker and one of the first eyewitnesses to be interviewed, remarked that it would have been busy that night around the Pont de Larrey, the principal road bridge across the canal.[2] Other witnesses reported seeing a woman, a man, and a child making their way along the canal path late in the evening. The wide expanse of the waterway and the cloud cover of a rainy night in midsummer would have eased the task of blending into the night's shades, a short distance from the road bridge, where the canal curves westward, obscuring the scene of the crime from that principal vantage point.[3]

The Dijon police were already looking for a missing child, five-year-old Henriette Barbey, who had disappeared shortly before noon the previous day. On 30 June, shortly after the body by the canal was found, her young classmate, Francine Barreau, told police officers that as the children were leaving school a woman "dressed all in black" had approached them. "Come with me," the woman had told Henriette. "Your mummy is at our house." Henriette had seemed to trust her abductor, giving her hand and following without protest.[4] Both girls attended the local *salle d'asile*, one of the nursery schools set up by the Catholic Church in urban areas to care for the young children of working women.[5]

A second witness, fourteen-year-old Louise Coquereaux, had been sent to fetch her niece from school that day and had recognized the as-yet unidentified woman. Coquereaux was not sure of her name, but they had occasionally worked alongside each other in the local tobacco factory, the Manufacture des tabacs.[6] Following Coquereaux's testimony, the police visited the factory foreman. He identified Marie-Françoise Fiquet, a thirty-one-year-old casual employee and known troublemaker, as the likely suspect.[7] On the morning of 30 June, the police went to her flat at 10 rue Musette and took her in for questioning.

The first press reports of the crime appeared on 1 July 1882. The principal regional paper, Dijon's *Le Bien Public*, devoted five days of coverage to the crime in its local news section. The *Bien Public* and another leading regional paper, *La Démocratie Bourguignonne*, stood politically to the moderate monarchist right and republican left of center, respectively, and both publications immediately expressed faith in the judiciary and the investigation.[8] On the first day of reporting, the *Démocratie Bourguignonne* printed the story of "a mysterious crime that has thrown our city into turmoil," noting that a suspect, the femme Fiquet, a "student midwife," had already been identified.[9]

On the evening of 1 July 1882, the *Bien Public* reiterated news reported that morning in *Le Petit Bourguignon*, the local left-wing popular daily newspaper:[10]

We read this morning in *Le Petit Bourguignon*:

> Since yesterday morning, there has been talk in the town of a mysterious event which has caused alarm in the neighborhood where the victim's family lives and which, pending the successful outcome of the investigation, suggests that the most monstrous crime has been committed. . . . On Thursday morning, at eleven o'clock, as the children were leaving the nursery school in rue Saint-Philibert, a woman is reported to have beckoned to little Henriette Barbey, aged five, whose parents live at 45 rue Berbisey.
>
> The child, thinking nothing of it, followed the unknown woman, who pretended that she had come to fetch her on behalf of her mother;

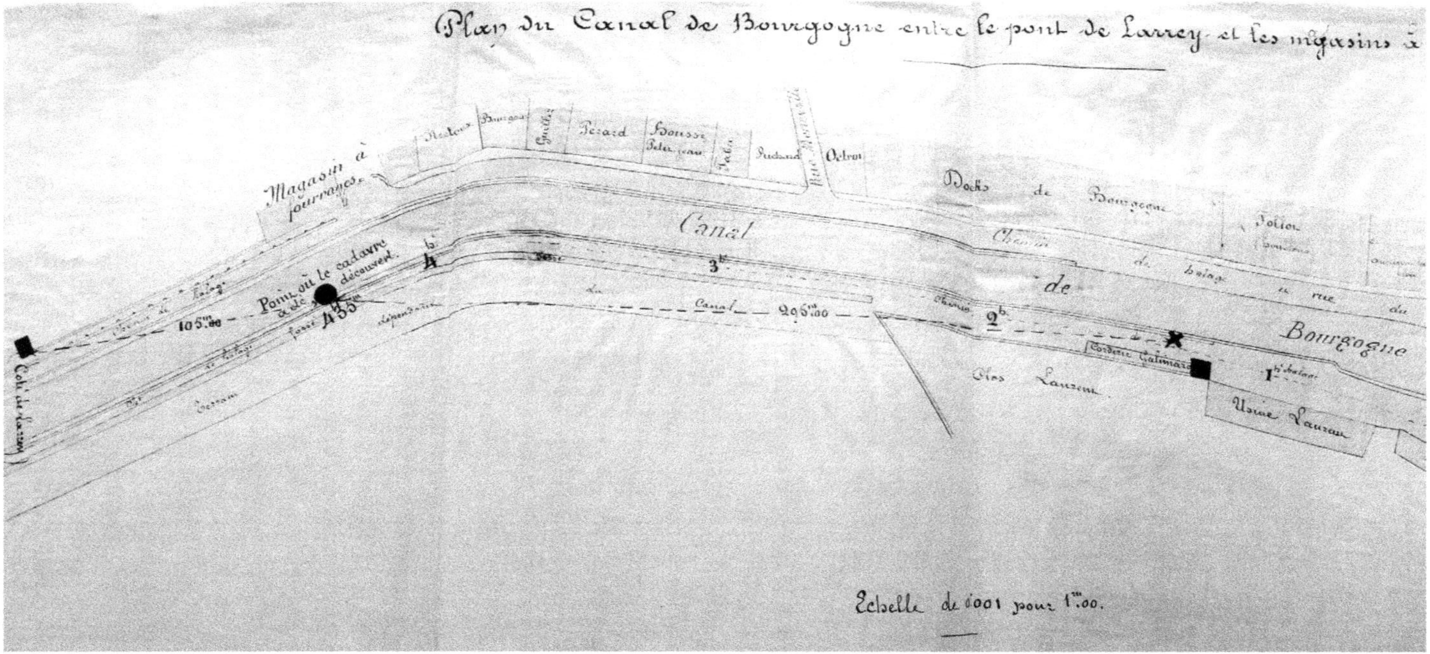

FIGURE 1A. Police map of the Canal de Bourgogne. Courtesy of the Archives Départementales de la Côte-d'Or in Dijon.

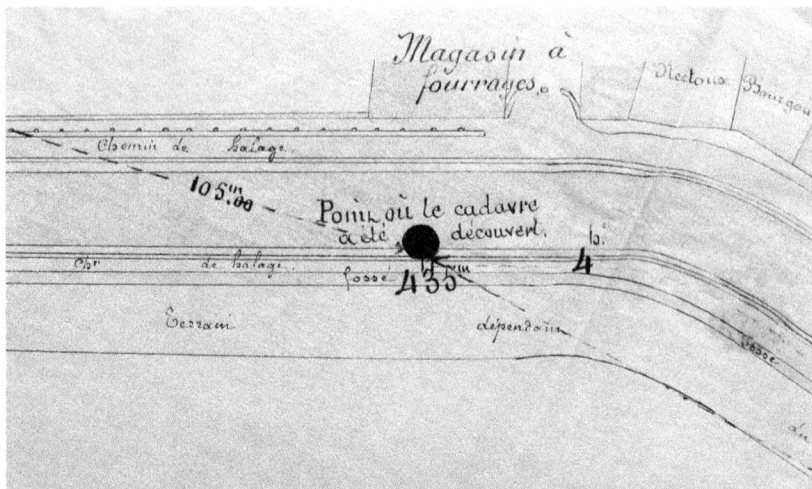

FIGURE 1B. The location of where Henriette Barbey's body was found on the police map of the Canal de Bourgogne. Courtesy of the Archives Départementales de la Côte-d'Or in Dijon.

but, alas, she would never be seen again. . . . In the afternoon, after having waited in vain until one o'clock, the parents' concern growing ever greater, they went to the school to find out what could have happened, and then to the home of their daughter's little friend. . . . The family spent the evening in a state of great anguish, for nothing had yet been discovered. It was not until yesterday morning that a workman, walking along the canal near the fodder suppliers, saw a girl child lying on the bank, and he went over to see what was wrong. Immediately he saw that the poor little girl was no more than a corpse.

Although the tone of the early coverage varied a little, to left and right Marie-Françoise Fiquet's culpability was assumed and expressed through simple narrative contrasts of guilt and innocence, darkness and light. These divisions were more pronounced in Dijon's proclerical and conservative publications, such as *Le Catholique* and *La Côte-d'Or*, but they were not absent from left-wing and center-left newspapers. The *Catholique* placed the crime in a broader social context and showed a primary concern with public morality, the integrity of the family, and the threat posed to society by the dysregulated "dangerous classes."[11] The publication drew on easily recognizable tropes of feminine evil, describing Fiquet as "a woman dressed in black . . . about whom grave suspicions are held," and contrasted her menacing image with that of the defenseless child victim, "the *unfortunate* Henriette Barbey,"

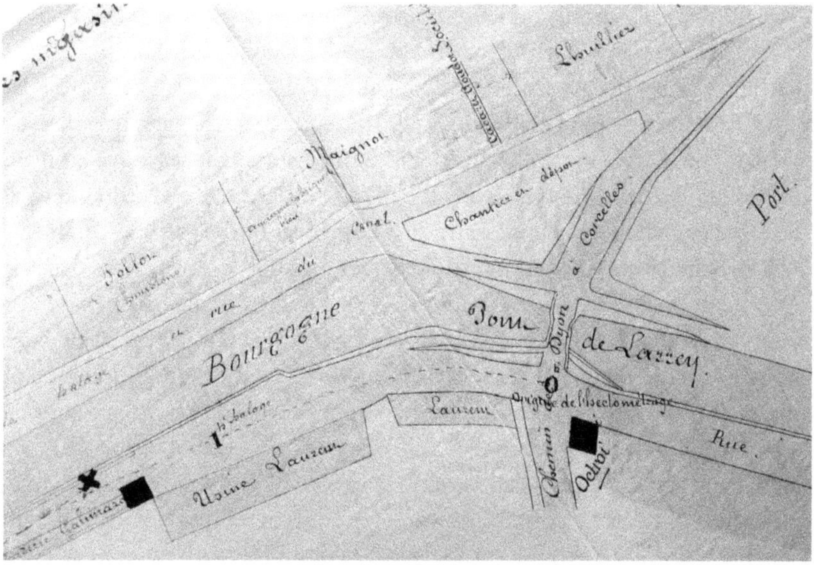

FIGURE 1C. The locations of key landmarks and eyewitness locations on the police map of the Canal de Bourgogne. Courtesy of the Archives Départementales de la Côte-d'Or in Dijon.

and "this *horrible* murder of a poor child."[12] The *Catholique* linked these events to a more generalized—but unspecified—anxiety about the corruption of innocent young children in French society: "In the last eight days alone, there have been three reports of attempted kidnappings of young children in similar circumstances."[13] These contrasts would be reasserted in later coverage of Henriette's funeral, attended by little girls dressed in white, carrying garlands of white flowers.[14]

In contrast, the moderate *Démocratie Bourguignonne* adopted a more circumspect tone from the start, reporting the same facts but omitting some of the speculatively emotive detail, such as the woman's black dress and the generalized sense of danger evoked by Henriette's murder.[15] Its reporting emphasized the poverty of the accused rather than her badness, calling her a "wretched woman," and expressed confidence that the mystery of this apparently senseless crime would be solved: "These motives will be revealed to us when the law has completed its investigations; but, until then, let us refrain from commenting."[16]

Some reports claimed that Henriette had been violently killed. The *Catholique* noted, "Her head was under the water and pressure marks on the sides of her head suggested that she had been violently restrained to suffocate her."[17] The *Progrès de la Côte-d'Or* described the injuries even more emphatically, as "strong pressure marks."[18] The autopsy report completed by Dr. Deroye a few days later would disprove these claims and concluded that Henriette's body seemed untouched: "There are no signs of violence or bruising on any part of the body."[19] These journalistic narrative choices, and perhaps early fictionalizations and embellishments, served the press's purpose of distorting and isolating the mundane details of the crime, such as the killer's black dress, to underline the uniqueness of the event and to locate a cause. The twentieth-century philosopher and historian Michel Foucault, who wrote extensively on crime and punishment, would later make the observation that, in the reporting of seemingly exceptional murders, such as the parricide Pierre Rivière, "it is necessary that all these little events— despite their frequency and monotony—appear as *singular, curious, extraordinary*, unique or almost unique in the memory of men."[20] The emphasis on the singularity of the criminal served a psychological distancing function: in this instance, to make an ordinary woman appear fundamentally different from her peers, even though she had more in common with them than could comfortably be admitted.

The investigation would quickly ascertain from various witnesses that the femme Fiquet had a notorious reputation as a fraud and a liar, a thief and a fornicator, and that she was a manipulative, attention-seeking morphine addict—a *morphinomane*. Further grave criminal suspicions would also weigh on her, and she would, in time, be accused of poisoning, carrying out clandestine abortions, and possibly infanticide. Although local people were shocked by Henriette's death, nobody was surprised to find that Marie-Françoise Fiquet was in the frame for the murder. Pierre Fiquet was also a suspect, but the nature and extent of his involvement was less obvious. The case was set to go to trial in December 1882 but was delayed several months due to a legal technicality. It finally went ahead in the early days of March 1883, and a verdict was reached on 8 March 1883.

Beyond the initial inquiries, the case hinged not on proving that the femme Fiquet had carried out this seemingly motiveless crime but on establishing the extent of her criminal responsibility.[21] How exactly did Henriette die, and when? Had she acted alone, or with her husband's assistance? If he was not an accomplice, why did he not try to save Henriette? What had motivated this young woman to commit such a cruel and cowardly act? Was she criminally responsible, or was she fully or partially insane? Finally, what role had her morphine addiction played in the story? This last question is key to the story.

Although opium had been used as an analgesic throughout the nineteenth century (and indeed for centuries before), morphine was a relatively new drug in 1882. Following the synthesization of morphine and the invention of the hypodermic syringe in the 1850s, morphine entered the medical mainstream in the 1870s.[22] The French government would impose greater controls on opiate prescriptions in 1916, but in the intervening period it was only controlled by pharmaceutical regulations designed to restrict access to poisons.[23] Most morphine users, like the femme Fiquet, were introduced to morphine by doctors; the addiction crisis was exacerbated by the exploitation of repeat prescriptions by unscrupulous pharmacists.[24] Yet, in France as in Britain, the disease model of drug addiction (in French *toxicomanie*) only began to emerge in the early decades of the twentieth century.[25] Uncertainty about the power of morphine over a subject's mind would become evident in the criminal proceedings in the Fiquet case, in which it was not deemed to be significant enough to excuse the crime, nor was it an indication of wider psychological disturbance in the criminal subject. Morphine use and abuse among the working classes in France had yet to be widely observed. Its profile as an upper-class drug was more clearly established in the United States and Europe, and Marie-Françoise Fiquet's case of problem morphine addiction was rare among her class.[26] She managed to gain access to opiates because she was utterly determined to seek out medical treatment at all costs, for a range of real and imagined disorders, and deployed her significant intellectual capacities to this end.

The investigation would gradually reveal a story that was both ordinary and extraordinary. A young psychiatrist, Dr. Marandon de Montyel, was tasked with observing Marie-Françoise Fiquet in the Chartreuse asylum in Dijon, where she was placed on 17 August 1882, six weeks after her arrest. Marandon noted early in his report that the suspect had spent time in hospitals in the region, at Besançon, Gray, and Épinal, where she had been treated for what transpired to be feigned physical and mental illnesses—for "extraordinary nervous symptoms."[27] After a long period of observation, the doctor concluded, "This affair remains a mysterious one, shrouded in darkness, that cannot be explained by either morphinomania, or nervous madness. If the motive was not due to sexual perversion, it is not any less unknown, and here there is a serious gap in the investigation that ought to make the expert circumspect in his conclusions when they may well lead to a death penalty."[28]

In this book, I consider the process via which the femme Fiquet's contemporaries reached the conclusions they did. The legal, medical, and journalistic narratives surrounding the affair reveal how dominant beliefs about class and gender norms intersected with the concepts of criminality and deviance in late nineteenth-century France. How was Marie-Françoise Fiquet judged by her peers and the society in which she lived? What did they think about her drug use and her manipulative and violent behavior? What account did Fiquet herself give of her actions, motives, and desires? What do the different elements of the story tell us about the culture and society in which its protagonists lived?

Today, in the twenty-first century, if a child is deliberately harmed by a female carer or other proxy, society is still shaken to the core by the breach of trust it represents. Such women, popularly termed "angels of death," are rarely treated leniently because they undermine the core assumptions many people hold about gendered human nature: As forensic psychologist Anna Motz has written, "the reality of women's violence is a truth too uncomfortable to take seriously: a taboo that offends the idealized notion of women as sources of love, nurture and care."[29] This taboo was also present in 1882, when contemporary ideologies of womanhood led to Fiquet being cast as a self-interested and monstrous killer.

Women who harm children have frequently exhibited what medical practitioners have since the early nineteenth century named "factitious" disorders. This is an umbrella term for feigned or induced illnesses, imposed on the self or others, and would later more commonly be known as Munchausen syndrome (and Munchausen by proxy). I shall argue that factitious disorder, or at least something resembling it, was at play in this criminal case; this is because Marie-Françoise Fiquet repeatedly harmed children and exhibited a long-standing obsession with clinical settings and medical treatments. The story of her young adult life brought together elements of a clinical picture of factitious disorder, including trauma and loss, female suffering, a desperate desire for recognition, and a disturbance of the maternal instinct.

The Fiquet case illustrates how factitious behaviors were beginning to be understood in the 1880s, the decade in which the father of psychoanalysis, Sigmund Freud, and the French neurologist Jean-Martin Charcot would define hysteria and begin to unpick the psychological mysteries of womanhood. Fiquet was viewed by her doctors as a "simulator" who shamelessly violated codes of virtuous, proletarian femininity and who was an exception to her class and gender. The evidence presented in this book, which only exists because the lives of the suffering poor came under state scrutiny when a terrible crime was committed, offers a window onto a time and a world in which the everyday pains and struggles of women's lives came to the fore when they transgressed these cultural codes. Fiquet attempted to give an account of her life and her motivations, and she revealed, I suggest, how her disordered behavior was rooted in a vague but persistent desire to exert control over the uncontrollable forces in her life, and indeed over life itself.

CHAPTER 1

Approaches

Following an initial examination of the available evidence, it became clear to me that the Fiquet affair merited scholarly attention as a case that contained clues to a deeper understanding of the lives of impoverished mothers in nineteenth-century provincial France. First, there was a fairly complete dossier of evidence pertaining to an unusually shocking killing that had never been studied before, as Foucault had found with the 1835 parricide Pierre Rivière.[1] Although we do not have the equivalent of Rivière's written memoir and confession, there was sufficient evidence to make the story more than just another *fait divers*, a small daily news item that titillates one day and is forgotten the next.[2] Second, although the Fiquet scandal cannot be considered a *grande affaire*, it did, like the Rivière case, test the limits of medicolegal knowledge and power. This is because, in a context in which many criminals were exonerated on psychiatric grounds, the femme Fiquet would be found responsible for her crime.[3] (As Philippe Artières has shown, the question of criminal responsibility dominated judicial and criminological debates in the last decades of the nineteenth century.)[4] Finally, the case offers a unique perspective on both the personal experience of addiction to morphine and the deployment of emergent knowledge about the drug in the late nineteenth century. It was also a test case that was cited in subsequent medical studies on the problem of morphine addiction in the general working population. There are many possible ways into the analysis of such a body of material: via medical history; the study of gender relations and female violence; the evolution of psychology and psychiatry; crime and punishment; and the interpretive lens of trauma and deviance. What follows is an overview of how these differing approaches might usefully converge in the study of the Fiquet affair.

Microhistory

We know from microhistorical scholarship, such as Natalie Zemon Davis's book on the revenant Martin Guerre, that because working people and peasants historically had limited literacy, they tended not to write self-revelatory documents. This was also true of nineteenth-century poor women, who would "become visible only when they meet the policymakers through their interactions in the public arena."[5] Public records, therefore, are useful, but they reveal little about people's feelings and personal experiences.[6] Documents in which people were required or forced to give an account of their lives, such as court records relating to criminal cases, are therefore precious sources.[7] For example, the inquisition registers from earlier periods in European history, mined (most famously) by Carlo Ginzburg and Emmanuel Le Roy Ladurie, offer such direct testimonies.[8] The recording of intimate behaviors revealed what motivated people; how they responded to crises; and their desires and ambitions, fears, and hopes for the future. Microhistory also achieves a unique perspective by focusing on the private sphere and on personal experiences of otherwise unknown actors from the past—often revealed only at moments of conflict and legal investigation.[9] Edward Berenson has attributed this shift to an "anthropological turn" in history, which "has enabled us to glimpse elements of religious belief, family life, sexual practices, and political power that we might otherwise have missed." This perspective helps us more reliably to reconstruct what people in the past thought about their fellow human beings, and how they judged them, both officially and unofficially.[10]

These more famous microhistorical studies have sparked lively discussion, at times, for ethical and methodological reasons. Can we really speak on behalf of people from subaltern classes? If we can, do we not risk replicating the power structures within which they were constrained—do we not ourselves become inquisitors? Similarly, in our desire to bring stories to life, is there a risk that we imagine a little too much, where the evidence is thin? And do we take the text at face value, without examining its rhetorical purpose or power? These critiques show, as does the present work, that any close reading of sources as narratives involves a level of personal engagement, interpretation, and individual emotional response that relies on the imagination (of the writer of history, and the reader) as well as the documented facts of the case.[11]

Women and Violence

There is a rich interdisciplinary research context into which this analysis of the Fiquet affair can be placed. The key scholarly interventions in the history of female violence and criminality in modern times have identified how women who kill have been represented in naturalistic and positivistic discourses as monstrous exceptions to the rules of "natural" femininity, of woman as wife, mother, and moral guardian.[12] Feminist scholars have countered this view by highlighting the "normality" of female criminals and even the relative banality of their actions, when understood in the context of the everyday stresses of their lives. Lisa Downing, for example, has argued that women who murder children are systematically treated as aberrations within patriarchal culture rather than as symptoms of it.[13] Anna Norris has contended that writings by incarcerated women have revealed the relevance of female suffering to crime; others maintain that female murderers found extraordinary and unorthodox solutions to common life stresses.[14]

Over the course of the nineteenth century, the number of women (proportional to men) being sent to prison in France gradually reduced, from 29 percent in 1830 to 15 percent in 1891, to only 6 percent by 1938. Yet, although cases of female violence were rare, they were often sensationalized and disproportionately impacted public opinion.[15] Michelle Perrot has argued that the female criminal is an idea as much as she is a physical reality, "thus the criminal woman is above all an image, a representation, a world of fantasy and imagination."[16] In line with this view, Ann-Louise Shapiro has shown that the perception of female criminality in fin-de-siècle France, as a statistically rare occurrence, was a cultural code that served as a foil for deeper societal anxieties. In the last decades of the nineteenth century, according to Shapiro, the cultural obsession with criminal women coincided with a decline in crimes committed by women: They made up only 14 percent of defendants (including women prosecuted for abortion and infanticide) and committed only 5.7 percent of homicides.[17]

Furthermore, Elissa Gelfand's research on the writing of female prisoners led her to observe some important patterns that pertain to the Fiquet case: "Crime in general was almost synonymous with poverty, and women's crime was synonymous with poverty, vagabondage, and prostitution. Patterns in female crime reveal it to be domestic or economic in nature. . . . It was therefore generally lower-class women who were arrested for crimes."[18] The Fiquet case conforms to this pattern, with the accused woman's life being affected by indigence, vagrancy, insecurity, sexual exploitation, and fragile health.

A common thread in these inquiries has been the critical appraisal of nineteenth-century criminology, notably Cesare Lombroso and Guglielmo Ferrero's obscurantist but influential tome, *La donna delinquente, la prostitua e la donna normale* (1893; translated into English in 1900 under the title *The Female Offender*), Raymond de Ryckère's *La femme en prison et devant la mort* (1898), and Camille Granier's *La femme criminelle* (1906).[19] Lombroso's vision of the typical female delinquent—inferior, calculating, and morally weak— was largely unchallenged in the contemporary criminological field, despite the Italian doctor's deterministic ideas being otherwise widely criticized.[20]

These authors' perspectives shared a view of woman as essentially weak and flawed, lacking the masculine virtues of courage and justice. These concerns generated "a convergence of anxieties about social disorder and cultural anarchy in the figure of the female criminal."[21] Female violence was a puzzle, because it went *against* the law of nature, according to which women, although the weaker sex, were supposed to be kind, gentle, and nurturing. Paradoxically, it also confirmed the view that, due to her moral and physical weakness, woman was more prone to scheming and debauchery.

There is nothing specifically feminist in questioning the idea of female criminal exceptionality, as this book aims to do, and as Foucault and André Gide have already done, in studies that have humanized the face of the violent criminal.[22] Indeed, Gide repeatedly mentioned his experience of "gêne," of feeling troubled, when looking a criminal in the face and seeing laid bare the unexceptionality of his or her life. This point is forcefully made in Gide's account of the Redureau affair. In Brittany in 1913, fifteen-year-old Marcel Redureau, an apparently docile and kind boy, brutally murdered seven members of the Mabit family. Gide suggested that murder can be arbitrarily and suddenly triggered, and while each investigation searches for an explanation that will reassure the public that killing is exceptional, the truth that often emerges is that it is the meaningless end point in a chain reaction. These accounts have in common the idea that the more we peer into these affairs, the less likely we are to find narrative closure, moral clarity, or sensation.[23] There is a tension, therefore, between the legal and journalistic pursuit of a rational explanation and the human frailty and mystery that sometimes marks violent crime, and which remains at the conclusion of the investigation.

A feminist consideration of the Fiquet affair ought to view it in the context of what we know about nineteenth-century French women, especially the indigent poor. Historians have noted that juries treated respectable bourgeois women, particularly those who committed crimes of passion, which typically involved a man and a woman in a couple, more leniently than working-class women, servants, and maids.[24] The more famous cases of Violette Nozière, who poisoned her parents, and the Papin sisters, domestic servants who sadistically murdered their employers, have shown that working-class female murderers in France could be judged severely.[25]

Juries and reporters had the capacity to be lenient, but their indulgence depended on how the defendant was expected to behave and how far she had veered from the path of virtue. Eliza Earle Ferguson has examined in detail how this played out in the courtroom, where working people described in detail the ins and outs of their daily lives, how women and men were expected to behave toward each other, and the instances in which violence was expected as opposed to when it was considered deviant.[26] Ferguson has shown that violent behavior was often understood and sometimes excused by the people who knew the victims and the perpetrators. The Fiquet affair, and similar cases, illustrated what happened when people were violent in ways that were not sanctioned or excused.

The trial of Madame Caillaux in 1914 was a case in point. Parisian socialite Henriette Caillaux shot and killed the editor of *Le Figaro* newspaper, Gaston Calmette, at point-blank range in his own office. The assassin believed that her husband, former French Prime Minster Joseph Caillaux, had been the victim of a smear campaign on the part of the press. Madame Caillaux attempted to convince a jury of her peers that hers, although clearly premeditated, was a crime of passion due to her overwhelming feminine emotions and being driven to act out of love for her husband. The prosecution case sought to prove the very opposite, that Madame Caillaux was guilty because she had dared to step outside of contemporary gender stereotypes and had acted like a man:

> A real woman does not . . . know how to use guns; a real woman does not practice marksmanship; and a real woman does not carry a loaded weapon in her handbag. *La femme, la vraie femme*, was for most French men of the era a creature governed by her emotions. Her intellect was limited, her practical and technical abilities restrained. The real woman acted not in the exterior world of politics and business, or even of literature and the arts, but in the inner sanctum of the home. She did not make a spectacle of herself—actresses, known for their sexual license, were not real women—nor did she seek to upstage her husband.[27]

Madame Caillaux could therefore be presented as a monster who, calculating and lacking in emotion in her violence, defied the laws of nature. Her defending attorney attempted to defeat this argument by making the case that Madame Caillaux had acted so recklessly precisely *because* of her feminine nature: She lacked self-possession and allowed herself to be entirely guided by emotions, not reason. Hers was a true crime of passion, even though it did not strictly fit the definition. The jury agreed, and Madame Caillaux was acquitted of all charges and walked free. The femme Fiquet's motives, by contrast, remained incomprehensible to her observers. How could anyone be driven to abduct and kill somebody else's child, for no reason at all?

The Fiquet case can be productively treated as a microhistory that illuminates some of the complex gender and class dynamics at play in late nineteenth-century French criminal cases. Fiquet was a woman who killed a child, and for this reason her observers were reluctant to consider *any* possible explanation for her behavior, even as they searched for a motive that could make a woman behave so unnaturally. Since Fiquet's crime took place at least partially within the home, the domain of feminine care and safety, her transgression was even more offensive to contemporary mores. Her own account, and her attempts to explain what motivated her, emerge only in the interstices of the wider story. It is, therefore, also instructive to consider the lacunae in the narrative that left the case unsatisfactorily resolved.

Nineteenth-century medical case histories, as Jan Goldstein has argued in the case of the hysteric-ecstatic Nanette Leroux, were particularly vivid in their novelistic detail, to the point of "unwittingly constituting the biographies of powerless people."[28] Medical and judicial records therefore lend themselves to microhistorical analysis. I would not suggest, however, that the femme Fiquet—who was an ambitious, ruthless, arch manipulator—was entirely powerless. These traits and her actions offered her some agency in a context of the economic and social limitations of her class and sex, and her personal vulnerability. Indeed, the Fiquet case challenges the commonplace that high-class, society courtesans were powerful and influential women in control of their lives, whereas poor working women (who also used occasional or regular prostitution to make money) were merely exploited victims.[29] We might compare Fiquet's resourcefulness to that of the demimondaine and sometime courtesan Meg Steinheil, who in 1908 was accused of killing her husband and mother and fabricating a cover story. In her testimony, Steinheil detailed how she exchanged social and political favors with friends and lovers for money—to maintain her family's standard of living. There was clearly give-and-take in both cases and common elements to the motivations of the two women.[30]

There is an important precedent in historical research for seeking to understand the cultural meaning of crimes. Fiquet's observers considered her actions inexplicable, and her motive unknowable. Yet, in anthropological terms, crimes always hold meaning because they necessarily entail interactions between human beings within a culture and the rupturing of a taboo within a social order. For example, Elizabeth Comack and Salena Brickey have argued from a sociological perspective that female violence is typically understood in terms of evil, madness, or victimhood. The first two positions are broadly reflected by nineteenth-century criminology and psychiatry, respectively. The final category of violent woman as the victim or product of patriarchy is an idea that emerged in the twentieth century. It is explicitly feminist and has been explored in depth by Downing and others, as previously mentioned. What is often more difficult to discern is "how women who use violence constitute themselves."[31] The scholars already mentioned have of course begun this work, and my intervention builds on that scholarship. This book is concerned with questions of narrative and representation, with how Marie-Françoise Fiquet's story was told and repeated, by herself and others, and what these retellings reveal about the lives of the working poor, and women's experiences within that class.

Factitious Disorders

Factitious disorder is a medical and psychiatric term used to describe the simulation of illness. It was first included in the third edition of the American *Diagnostic and Statistical Manual of Mental Disorders* in 1980 (DSM-III), and in the tenth edition of the *International Statistical Classification of Diseases* (ICD-10, 1990), the manual published by the World Health Organization and recognized in French psychiatry.[32] In French-language psychiatric manuals, factitious disorders are named "troubles factices" or "pathomimies," and due to the enduring influence of psychoanalysis in France and hostility to the Anglo-American medical traditions, as we shall see, the ICD classifications are preferred.[33]

The 2013 DSM-5 applies the label to people who "falsify illness in themselves or in another person, without any obvious gain."[34] It is an attention-seeking behavior seen as distinct from malingering and hypochondria, which have more obvious motives. Factitious disorders have, at the extreme end of the spectrum, been labeled as Munchausen syndrome, or Munchausen by proxy (when inflicted on another, such as a child).[35] This clinical description is also used in France ("le syndrome de Münchhausen" and "le syndrome de Münchhausen par procuration"). The disorder is often identified within health care settings in which perpetrators can act out their desires, and it can lead to serious harm, even death.[36]

These disturbances are, according to some hypotheses, causally linked to the early experience of psychological trauma, neglect, and abandonment.[37] Others maintain that they are better described as personality disorders linked to pathological grandiosity and ambition and that they are motivated by a craving for recognition that may or may not be linked to trauma. The desire to inflict harm and pain on others can appear inexplicable, and some people kill simply for the pleasure of killing or for the feeling of power it confers on them.[38] These two explanations are not, of course, mutually exclusive, and elements of the Fiquet case fit both frameworks. The femme Fiquet's simulated illnesses and the harm she inflicted on others, as we shall see, were connected to ruthless ambition and a desire to exert power and control over her own personal circumstances, and to exploit the weak.

Most historical records of simulated illness go back to antiquity and the early Christian era. Such stories have been a source of alarm and amusement through history and have often been fictionalized and dramatized—for example, in Molière's 1673 play *Le Malade imaginaire*. In modern times, factitious disorders were first described in medical literature in 1838, in the Scottish physician Hector Gavin's treatise on malingering soldiers and sailors, *On Feigned and Factitious Diseases*. Crucially, however, Gavin noted various subtypes within his schema whose motives went beyond malingering. These "patients" gained gratification from their deceit and seemed primarily motivated by attracting compassion and attention from clinicians rather than evading military service.[39]

In the French psychological sciences, simulated illnesses have also been observed since the early nineteenth century. The treatises tended to focus, like the English-language ones, on occupational malingering, but they also broached the simulation of madness, self-inflicted wounds, faked suicide and death, and "mania" for unnecessary surgeries.[40] In *Des maladies simulées et des moyens de les reconnaître* (1870), Edmond Boisseau offered a comprehensive survey of the different illnesses that could be feigned but did not specifically mention simulation for attention or gratification.[41] Arguably, the medicolegal reports on the Fiquet affair constituted, as we shall see, a contribution to this literature that bridged these earlier descriptions of malingering and simulated illness and later appraisals of Munchausen syndrome by proxy.

Between these early nineteenth-century descriptions of feigned illness and the more specific (and rather waspish) descriptions of Munchausen syndrome in 1951 by Richard Asher and Munchausen by proxy in 1977 by pediatrician Roy Meadow, there were observations of hysteria in the 1880s and 1890s on which the early twentieth-century insights of psychoanalysis were built. The role of suggestion was central to the conceptualization of hysteria, as was the possibility that patients could be motivated by unconscious "secondary gain" from assuming the sick role.[42] It was not, therefore, a completely new idea when Asher gave the syndrome a name. The prominence of the diagnosis in the twentieth century and apparent increase in cases has been interpreted in the context of the professionalization of medicine in the nineteenth century followed by the emergence of universal health care provision in Britain and France after the Second World War. Increased access to treatment, coupled with the medicalization of life stages that had previously been ritualized in nonmedical ways, provided a fertile context for factitious disorders and consequent power struggles between doctors and patients to occur.[43] As other scholars have noted on the emergence of nostalgia as a clinical diagnosis, the early to mid-nineteenth century was a period when common human problems, in this case, literally "homesickness," came to be framed increasingly as medical dilemmas with specific treatments. In contrast with factitious disorder, nostalgia went on to be naturalized as a human feeling rather than a perversion or disease.[44]

Historians of medicine tend to resist the retrospective diagnosis of illness because knowledge is always situated within its own time and the process risks being anachronistic. Rigid adherence to this idea, however, can also result in frustratingly circular analyses. For example, Chris Millard has argued that the emergence of Munchausen syndrome was closely imbricated with developments in twentieth-century sociology and anthropology, related to the importance of social setting in understanding disease.[45] For this reason, Millard argues, we cannot apply the syndrome across time. The problem with this view, and with medical historians' general rejection of the consideration of early manifestations of disorders yet to be formally clinically described, is that it implies an exaggeratedly rigid break between the later nineteenth century and the early twentieth century. The sociological and anthropological models of the 1930s through the 1950s did not emerge in a vacuum, and the democratization of access to medical treatment was not something that suddenly occurred after the Second World War.

Millard's argument draws on the philosopher of science Ian Hacking's concept of "making up people." Hacking has argued that certain illnesses are brought into being through the process of being observed, described, and named. For example, multiple personality disorder (later named dissociative identity disorder), Hacking argues, "as an idea and as a clinical phenomenon was invented around 1875." The creation of a diagnosis "creates new ways for people to be" and has, he suggests, an impact on the subjective experience of illness/disorder and interactions with other people—family, friends, employers, and so on.[46] But, crucially, Hacking does admit that there are exceptions to this claim about the temporal limits of diagnosis. He allows that there are "a very few earlier examples" that are later reinterpreted as being cases of—following his example—multiple personality disorder. This supports my argument, which is that the Fiquet affair can legitimately be viewed as a diagnostic forerunner. Similarly, Hacking admits that certain clusters of symptoms or acts (such as fugues, or strange wandering behavior) may be observed throughout time but that they only come into being as actual *illnesses* when they are diagnosed as such, at a particular point in time, by a clinician.[47]

Hacking's idea concerns what he has termed *transient mental illness*—disorders that seem to exist only in certain places and times. These are culture-bound syndromes that in the era of modern clinical practice have been medicalized. The case can be made that Munchausen syndrome was similarly "produced" in the 1950s in the UK and was generalized to other Western countries in the decade that followed. But Hacking has also said, "I do not believe there is a general story to be told about making up people. Each category has its own history."[48] The peculiarity of Munchausen syndrome is that it is partly characterized by a lack of insight and a concerted attempt to simulate illness where it does not exist. A further strangeness in this instance is that the diagnosis of Munchausen's is itself an absence, apart from the disorder. In other words, it is the opposite of a diagnosis of illness; it is the detection of a fraud and the absence of real disease. This circularity explains why Munchausen syndrome has never been called an illness, and it fits more closely the concept of personality disorder that would evolve later in the twentieth century.

As we shall see in the Fiquet case, early elements of a new, democratized medical infrastructure were beginning to be rolled out in the later nineteenth century. As medical technologies and treatments evolved, state-backed services began to serve the poorer urban populations of cities. Fiquet availed herself of these services liberally and managed to sustain her morphine addiction in part through free prescriptions and the availability of syringes. Richard Kanaan and Simon Wessely have also shown that the idea of "assuming the sick role" for secondary gain had been recognized by Charcot in the 1880s, and subsequently by Pierre Janet, Freud, and Karl Menninger in the early decades of the twentieth century, as part of the clinical picture of hysteria. Hysterics were by definition not "really" ill, so malingering or factitious disorders could similarly be considered illnesses in themselves.[49] Contemporary clinical literature in France has overtly embraced the psychoanalytical legacy of this approach, placing neuroses and "perversions" under the umbrella of personality disorders, as behaviors that are not-quite-mad but not-quite-normal either.[50]

It is significant that the Fiquet affair occurred in Dijon, with a medical observation in Paris, in the early 1880s. This was before emerging theories of hysteria were fully developed and made public—Charcot's clinical lessons were published at the end of the decade, and Freud and Breuer's influential work, *Studies on Hysteria*, was published in 1895.[51] The femme Fiquet's distress and supposed illness was treated with great skepticism and little sympathy. Importantly, in their reports, her doctors did *not* consider her to be a genuine hysteric but a false one, and her simulations were labeled fraudulent rather than as manifestations of illness. Her case therefore fell between two important historical moments in the background to diagnosing factitious disorders, as summarized by Kanaan and Wessely: "The history of hysteria can be argued to show not a steady decline into stigmatizing malingering, but a base of suspicion and disregard from which it was briefly raised by the support of Charcot and Freud; a period of respectability, even popularity, that has fallen away as their authority crumbled."[52]

Marie-Françoise Fiquet was treated harshly because the clinicians who observed her had no available explanatory model with which to make sense of her behavior and her dark motivations. However, this model was emerging, and the twentieth-century conceptualization of factitious disorders had deep roots in the nineteenth century. In particular, the insights of psychoanalysis, and psychodynamic therapeutic models, which originated in the 1880s and evolved under the influence of nineteenth-century medicine, offer a compelling cultural explanation for what have often been viewed as inexplicable behaviors.

This view is illustrated by French psychoanalyst Caroline Eliacheff, who begins her 2005 article on Munchausen syndrome by proxy by noting the "unusually vitriolic tone" and obvious attitude of "animosity" shown by Asher and Meadow in their clinical descriptions of disordered patients. Eliacheff argues that Meadow's description of the toxic coupling of bad mothers with complicit doctors was fundamentally misleading, and one that led to miscarriages of justice. She suggests, rather, that Munchausen by proxy warrants a psychodynamic explanation to identify the traumatic root of the disorder—doctors should be diagnosing, not detecting.[53]

In France, the diagnostic picture for factitious disorders was complicated by the fact that the 1950s and 1960s were decades during which levels of trust between clinicians and families were low, and the authority of diagnosing doctors began to be challenged. This has been more clearly evidenced by historians through the case of autism treatment in France, where psychoanalytical explanations and treatments for the disorder dominated clinical theory and practice for longer than in comparable countries. These ideas assumed that parents, especially mothers, caused the appearance of autism in their children through a lack of emotional engagement with their infants. In the later 1960s, French parents began to reject this bleak diagnosis and sought alternative approaches to caring for their children. This would suggest that, *pace* Eliacheff, doctors' suspicions toward mothers and the belief that they could seriously harm their children was as prevalent in France as elsewhere.[54]

Contemporary responses to the events surrounding Henriette Barbey's death at the hands of the femme Fiquet show that some of the same dilemmas and tensions were present: The investigation sought to establish how much Fiquet's actions could be attributed to mental disease, drawing on the concepts of hysteria and mania, and how much to criminal and immoral tendencies. The medical professionals called on to assess Fiquet explicitly described her behavior as "simulation" of illness, and they attributed it to attention-seeking tendencies: They thus offered many of the diagnostic elements of the latterly identified disorder, and they shared Asher's and Meadow's distrust of the alleged "patient." What contemporary doctors did not posit, and what psychodynamic explanations suggest, was a connecting thread between the simulation of illness, personal ambition and grandiosity, obsession with medicine, trauma and loss, and female violence.

The description of factitious disorders offers us a mutating medical model, therefore, via which we might make cautious conceptual links between events in Fiquet's case history, the account she gave of her crime, and later (but not very much later) psychological theories relating to Munchausen syndrome. Today, for example, we might view the femme Fiquet's violence as rooted in the personal trauma of infant loss.[55] Alternatively, since she could not accept her own ordinariness and believed she was an important person who had been overlooked, Fiquet perhaps sought to make her life significant through notoriety and the addictive thrill of killing. Her behavior might therefore be viewed through the lens of personality disorder rather than trauma.

In this book, I demonstrate that Marie-Françoise Fiquet suffered from a generic factitious disorder that she imposed on herself and other victims. Hers was an extreme case of disturbance that would later be clinically described as Munchausen syndrome. In discussing the case, therefore, it would be historically inaccurate to suggest that Fiquet literally *had* Munchausen syndrome, a diagnosis that was not available to her examining doctors; nor, to put it in Hacking's terms, was it a "way to be a person," or a coherent subjective experience that it was possible to have in 1882.[56] Nevertheless, Fiquet did exhibit all the elements of an extreme factitious disorder that led to poisoning and murder, and as such we should consider hers an early case in an emerging epidemiological paradigm.

Trauma, Perversion, and Psychodynamic Models of Distress

There are only two possible explanations for factitious disorders, and variations of these have been leveraged in observations of such cases from the early nineteenth century to the present. The first is that factitious disorders are the result of trauma that in turn produces a destructive repetition compulsion. This idea was offered by Freud in his 1923 essay "Beyond the Pleasure Principle" to explain why some people are compelled to keep repeating behaviors that cause harm to themselves and others. Freud suggested that the compulsion to repeat was rooted in a desire to gain mastery over a difficult and uncontrollable experience—prototypically, the experience of an infant being abandoned by his or her mother.[57]

The second is that these disorders occur spontaneously and can only be explained by the presence of evil in the human soul or motivated by secondary gain that cannot be explained by trauma (for example, a thrill experienced by harming and killing, or a feeling of satisfaction gained from medical attention). Psychoanalytical theory is the only model of human motivation that can encompass both these explanations and contain the inherent instability of the concept of trauma. The connecting elements are the desire for control and mastery, the concepts of the life and death drives, and the idea of perversion.[58]

The original meaning of the Greek word *trauma* is a physical wound, and Freud's concept of "traumatic neurosis" also gave it a psychological meaning. Some cultural critics, such as Cathy Caruth, view trauma as a universal term that applies to recurring suffering that cannot be articulated, only witnessed.[59] Others, such as Ruth Leys, counter this view with the argument that, genealogically speaking, trauma is an idea that holds an "irruptive character," recurring at different historical moments and mutating through time.[60] Leys's approach challenges those medical historians who, in their critiques of retrospective diagnosis, presuppose the linear development of medical concepts. Leys's idea that trauma was understood in the nineteenth century by Charcot as essentially mimetic—involving an imitation of, or identification with, the original aggressor—is very persuasive in the case of the femme Fiquet, who, I suggest, killed a child because her own children died. Death was a force that initially lay beyond her control and which she sought to bring under her own influence.[61]

The psychoanalytical concept of the repetition compulsion is taken seriously in psychiatry, perhaps because it is so evident in so many disorders, even where other Freudian concepts are considered discredited. For example,

Harold Kaplan and Benjamin J. Sadock offer the following informative summary of how psychoanalysis informs psychiatry in the understanding of factitious disorders:

> Psychodynamic theories have focused on the concepts of mastery, masochism, and mothering. Striving for mastery may especially apply to factitious disorder patients with predominantly psychological signs and symptoms. . . . Because many patients with factitious physical symptoms seem to have suffered traumatic illnesses as children, adult factitious illness behavior may represent an attempt to master and to feel in control of situations in ways in which they never did as children. They demand or refuse procedures and leave the hospital against medical advice when they feel they are losing control.[62]

Kaplan and Sadock claim that factitious patients are affected by masochism and might be compelled to relive an abusive relationship by positioning doctors and other carers as "symbolic parents." When imposed on others, factitious disorders are to some extent sadistic, "a *perversion of mothering* in which a child is dehumanized by the mother and instead serves as a fetishized object through which the mother's dependency needs are met."[63] This could be benign and limited to moments of helicopter parenting, or, taken to its extreme, it could lead to mothers seriously harming and even murdering children.

Perversion is also a concept that is taken seriously in French psychiatry. To identify "perversion" in human behavior, in a psychiatric context, is not necessarily to offer the sort of value judgment it would typically carry in common parlance. It is, rather, a descriptive term to convey the potential of all human instincts to be directed away from their original biological or evolutionary purpose. Perversion can be the sexualization of trauma, in the broadest sense. It does not necessarily relate to the physical sex act but to the drives, to libido, and to human instinct and desire. In the case of the maternal instinct, we would normally expect it to produce nurturing behavior, with the child drawing energy from the mother. But if that instinct is perverted it leads to the mother (or the woman standing in for the mother) parasitically feeding off a dependent child to satisfy her own needs.

Factitious disorders are one of the most significant sources of female violence. On the one hand, we tend to accept that male violence is inevitable and sometimes even necessary; we may seek to mitigate its effects, but we cannot eliminate it. Female violence, on the other hand, seems unnecessary and unnatural and is therefore difficult to accept, as inevitable as it *also* is—

especially when connected to the mothering role. As befits this picture, and as we discover through the close examination of the sources, Marie-Fran-çoise Fiquet lost at least two babies and was accused of killing other infants and vulnerable adults when carrying out paramedical procedures. She was fixated on the idea of becoming a midwife, an occupation that was quickly being medicalized and professionalized, and this provided fertile ground for the growth of her factitious disorder. The love Fiquet perhaps felt for her lost infants turned to hatred, nurture turned to destruction, and libidinal satisfaction was taken in harming and killing because it was something over which she could exert control. It is also possible that her destructive urges preexisted the deaths of her babies and might have produced the violence that, according to another interpretation, could be read as the result of trauma.

I shall argue that Marie-Françoise Fiquet's own account of her actions is built around a central control paradox.[64] In the telling of her story, she expressed a recurring desire to control the forces of life and death. According to this interpretation, killing was the perverse solution she brought to the problems of pain, loss, grief, and the wretched brutality and perceived insignificance of her life. Yet, paradoxically, in attempting to control these elements of her life, Fiquet's actions reeled out of control and her urges came to be curtailed by a society that needed to contain her and had little interest in understanding what drove her.

Representations

Dominique Kalifa has observed that crime is almost always "an incomprehensible event" and that "the intelligibility of crime seems only to occur through its representation."[65] This book is based on the close, narrative analysis of these various "representations" with the aim of isolating Marie-Fran-çoise Fiquet's experiences as a poor woman, a morphine user, and a killer. It also aims to understand clearly how she fitted into the world in which she lived—what kind of life she had, and what other people thought of her and her actions. My approach to the case is based on close readings of the available documents as texts in historical context.

The case would become a stage on which competing systems of knowledge and visions of human nature were rehearsed: The legal system sought to establish who was responsible for her crime; the medical experts pondered the extent to which the accused woman's drug addiction and mental disturbance affected her judgment; and the press sought to offer a simple and coherent narrative of good and evil, and to reassure the public of the definitive exclusion of this aberrant element from their community.[66]

What follows is structured and presented chronologically (as far as possible) according to when the information emerged. Chapters 2 and 3 present the early press reports from July 1882 and analyze them alongside the *dossier de procédure* in some depth, with a focus on the first pieces of information that appeared. This included Fiquet's shifting and fragmented account of her own actions, thoughts, and experiences. The multivocal quality of the archive material means that the dossier produces the most chaotic, conflicting, and uncertain version of the story. It does, however, reveal miscellaneous details about the lives of the protagonists that were suppressed in later iterations of the narrative but which are of great interest to this book. Chapter 4 focuses on the medical reports commissioned by the investigation. The reflections of the femme Fiquet's psychiatrists were the first attempt to construct a coherent account of the case and to impose a provisional medical frame onto an inexplicable event. Chapter 5 considers the final "representation" of events through the reporting of the trial in the regional press, and chapter 6 draws together the threads of the story by considering the afterlives of its main characters as well as some information that came to light after its conclusion. I consider two parallel cases that raise pertinent questions in an interlude between chapters 4 and 5.

The archive emerges out of the disorder of the world, and the piecemeal investigation of Fiquet's crime does not offer a complete picture of the people whose lives it records.[67] I can only present a plausible hypothesis to explain what drove Fiquet and why she acted as she did; at times this will mean working in what Ginzburg has called that "intermediate zone, pointing to historical possibility ('what might have been') and not hard evidence."[68] In the process, as Arlette Farge urges all historians to do, I must make the case for telling *this* story, and for why it matters, because of how "each individual constructed her own agency out of what history and society put at her disposal."[69]

My focus in analyzing the Fiquet dossier is on the complexities within the ordinary, in a case where most sides agreed that they could not determine a motive and in which the mystery of female life for its would-be interpreters remained. Together, these documents offer a rich seam of material that provides collected information about the everyday lives of the people of Dijon, the specific ways in which women bore their sufferings, and children who were at risk of harm. It is a general story about these struggles, but it is also a unique case of psychic rupture, of how life went wrong for one woman, in one place, at one point in history.

The Fiquet case offers disturbing evidence of the possible "naturalness" of female violence—of how easy it is to quietly kill, how addictive it can be to control who lives and who dies. Marie-Françoise Fiquet spoke repeatedly of her need to cede to this impulse, to satisfy a deep craving. In carrying out her actions she achieved a state of pleasure and satisfaction, temporarily perhaps, that took her far away from her pain. But it was also a wound to which she was compelled to return.

CHAPTER 2

The Investigation

Dijon today is a visually unchanging city due to its rich, protected architectural heritage, but its dynamism over the past two centuries has been equally impressive. Today, it is proud to call itself a "Green City," in which the grand town squares have been transformed from dingy car parks into bright, pedestrian, shared civic zones, connected by a network of accessible, sleek tramways. The beginning of this long process of dynamic modernization was underway by the early 1880s, and the local population was in flux.

Dijon had been a commercially and politically significant city since the period of the Grand Duchy of Burgundy, in the ninth to the fifteenth centuries. It was capital of both the administrative *département* of La Côte-d'Or and the historic region of Burgundy (Bourgogne). By 1882, in common with many French towns, Dijon was growing and industrializing rapidly. The 1881 census recorded a population of 55,453—up from 42,573 the previous decade.[1] In 2019, the population had reached 158,002, and today it is the seventeenth-largest city in France.[2] It grew bigger still after the 1870–71 Franco-Prussian War, due to the emigration of people from Alsace and Lorraine, territories annexed by a newly unified Germany. The city's industries and new railways offered opportunities for these migrant workers.

In the nineteenth century, the city began manufacturing the signature food products for which it became famous, *la moutarde de Dijon* and *la crème de cassis*—a sweet, dark, black currant liqueur. The wider Burgundian region was one of the most important wine-producing provinces in the world; due to its thriving economies in essential and luxury foods and drink, the region was prosperous, and the city enjoyed a rich cultural heritage.

Pierre Gras's history of the city, published in 1981, celebrates several nineteenth-century innovations, such as the establishment of the Lycée and the new university Faculties of Science, Letters and Medicine (1805–9); the opening of the Canal de Bourgogne (1832); the first uses of gas lighting in the 1840s; the incremental construction of railways, sidewalks, and public fountains; the opening of the girls' public high school (1897); and the first general electric power distribution in the 1880s. According to contemporary antiquarian and chronicler of the city Henri Chabeuf, the establishment of scholarly institutions reinvigorated the city in the years after the Revolution, and pioneering engineer Henry Darcy enabled the radical modernization of Dijon in his creation of a network of water fountains in 1839–40.[3]

These developments meant that by the 1850s, Dijon was no longer "a third-rate, quiet and empty town," with a static or slightly declining population; it was rapidly becoming a vibrant city of modernity. The streets were paved and transportation was modernized. Fifteen years after the Fiquet affair, in 1897, Chabeuf would write, "Dijon has changed more in twenty-six years than it has in centuries."[4] The 1880s were the apex of this dramatic transformation, and the significance of the Fiquet affair must be appreciated in this context.

Marie-Françoise Fiquet and her family, like many poorer working people from the surrounding regions, were drawn to Dijon to work in its factories. The Dijon Manufacture des tabacs opened in 1876 and employed more than five hundred local workers, most of them women. In the nineteenth and twentieth centuries, these factories were still government run (the French tobacco industry had been a state monopoly since the ancien régime). Today, such factory buildings, where they survive, form an important part of France's industrial architectural heritage. Every major French city had a tobacco factory until the last remaining one, in the Auvergne city of Riom, closed in 2017. The exodus from country to city and the immense societal, architectural, and technological changes that occurred over the course of the nineteenth century have been reflected in the work of canonical French authors such as Émile Zola and Charles Baudelaire, who depicted both the dynamism of the nineteenth-century city and the experiences of poverty and alienation they created. Rural life remained harsh, but conditions in cities were challenging in different ways. Many families lived in tiny apartments, and working people were often forced to exist in insalubrious conditions.

Most went without electricity, gas, and running water well into the twentieth century. Public fountains were the main source of clean water, and cooking and heating were provided by open fires or wood-fueled stoves. Winters in central France are bitterly cold and bleakly dark, and even in turn-of-the-century Paris only one house in ten was connected to a sewer system. Urban hygiene was an urgent social question, with larger European cities such as Geneva being metaphorically imagined as squalid, swarming anthills or personified as leprous bodies.[5]

However, city life also brought newfound freedoms for working people, including women. Prostitutes had long been seen as "public women" who walked the streets, but other groups of women increasingly inhabited social spheres outside the home. As Elizabeth Wilson has argued, "The very presence of unattended—unowned—women constituted a threat both to male power and to male frailty. Yet although the male ruling class did all it could to restrict the movement of women in cities, it proved impossible to banish them from public spaces. Women continued to crowd into the city centers and the factory districts." The documents in the Fiquet affair dossier show, in some detail, how the accused woman inhabited the city in which she lived; how she moved around it, autonomously, pleasing herself, in some contrast to the type of social policing to which upper-class women would have been subjected.

The Main Actors

The femme Fiquet lived in a small, unkempt apartment on the top floor at 10 rue Musette—a busy street on the western edge of central Dijon—with her husband, Pierre, and their thirteen-year-old daughter, Marie-Louise (known as Louise). Louise had been born out of wedlock, fathered by an unknown man, and legally acknowledged by Pierre Fiquet as his daughter. The investigation soon learned that the femme Fiquet had worked at the factory alongside the dead girl's mother, Olympe Barbey. Henriette's aunt, the widow Barbey, was also a neighbor of the Fiquet family in the same rue Musette building, which was just a ten-minute walk from the rue Berbisey, where the victim's family lived. Although their lives intersected geographically, both the Barbeys and the Fiquets insisted that they had never met.

According to the *Démocratie Bourguignonne*, when arrested and questioned, the femme Fiquet denied having anything to do with Henriette's death. Taken to view the child's body, she appeared callously indifferent to the sight of it:

The femme Fiquet countered [the claims of the two witnesses] with the most emphatic denials. Despite this, she was taken to prison. The

police went to her home, and after a meticulous search, they soon discovered the victim's earrings, her comb, and the paper in which the
cherries she had given the child to eat were wrapped. Yesterday morning the femme Fiquet was taken to the victim, but she refused to look
at the poor child, lying dead on her bed.[6]

Later that day, Fiquet would accuse her husband, who had only recently
returned home after a spell in hospital, of committing the crime. Following her denunciation, Pierre Fiquet was also arrested, and he would subsequently be tried alongside his wife for Henriette's murder.

The French "inquisitorial" legal system is guided by the Napoleonic Code
(civil and criminal codes) and can be distinguished from the "adversarial"
system of common-law jurisdictions such as the United States and England.
French criminal investigations were not primarily a police affair. Although
the police worked with the investigation, especially in the early stages, the
process was overseen from the beginning by the French public prosecution
service, called *le parquet*, headed up by an investigating magistrate, the *juge
d'instruction*, whose role was to inquire into the facts rather than to arbi-
trate between two advocates in court. Other features of the French system
included the use of "confrontations" in which key witnesses and the defendants were brought together to face each other's accusations and denials, and
rather loose rules of evidence, as we shall see.

Following the first reading of the indictment in the assizes court, in
December 1882 the *Progrès de la Côte-d'Or*, a republican center-right newspaper, reported that Marie-Françoise Fiquet's defense lawyer, Étienne Metman, had expressed concern that in the months from the original crime in
July to when the defendants came to trial in December, "public opinion had
been much too preoccupied with this affair." The *Progrès* responded, "Is it to
be hoped, then, that we should stay silent on the subject of this monstrous
crime?"[7] Indeed, the primary strategy adopted by the press in the days and
weeks following Henriette's murder had been a Manichean one, to define
the ways in which the femme Fiquet could be singled out as a malevolent
killer and an exception to her sex and class, the embodiment of pathological
femininity.

In the days following the discovery of Henriette's body, in early July
1882, the conservative press repeatedly pushed the image of the mysterious
"woman in black," initially invoked by Henriette's young classmate, Francine
Barreau. In French, the black queen chess piece is called "la dame noire," an
image that carries connotations of ruthlessness and erotic power. Out of
the available evidence the press was able to begin constructing a culturally

recognizable, if somewhat one-dimensional, picture of a monstrous, seductive woman-who-kills—a femme fatale. In inhabiting this stereotype, Fiquet was also presented as transgressing class boundaries by moving from the anonymous working classes into the demimonde, even if only partially, or in the public imagination.

The significance of the "dame noire" or femme fatale image is extensive. It was an important cultural trope in the later nineteenth century, born from French Decadence. It expressed a primal fear of sexually potent and calculatedly manipulative women. The archetypally alluring woman was often imagined as a mythical animal or monster—for example, a sphinx who coolly seduced and killed or a vampire who parasitically drained the energy of her lovers. The contemporary iconography of the femme fatale was also recognizable. Such woman-as-sphinx imagery was popular with the Symbolists, such as Belgian painter Fernand Khnopff, who depicted the creature with a contemporary woman's head and the body of a wild cat.[8] The chilling sphinx was inviting and familiar but also ruthless and impervious to her victim's suffering; she also represented a phallic, virilized woman, underscoring the power of female sexual desire.[9] As Mireille Dottin-Orsini has noted, the femme fatale was above all the "woman who is fatal *to men*."[10]

She was often associated with serpents, with Eve representing the Fall and the corruption of man by woman. Snake imagery reflected contemporary religious doubts about whether women had souls. These questions about the humanity of women were also present in the evocation of the vampire, an image that in the later nineteenth century came to be associated with emancipated women.[11] Significantly, for cultural critic Bram Dijkstra, "The sphinx . . . still had the outward appearance of the warm, all-yielding mother . . . a promise of benevolent passivity."[12] This duplicitous appeal also applied to the female murderer, who promised comfort but delivered destruction.

This emerging fiction of course had some basis in truth. Even as Fiquet's motive seemed inexplicable, it seemed clear to reporters from the outset that she had lured a child to her home and caused her death, and the investigation at times wondered whether the motive had been sexual. The facts of the case were painstakingly gathered in the months between the arrest of the femme Fiquet and her husband in July and the first court hearing in December 1882. The one-dimensional picture of a ruthless child killer who inhabited "public opinion" was the result of the distillation and drip-dripping of information to the press that occurred over the course of those months.

The contents of the *dossier de procédure* were gathered to gain as many different perspectives on the Fiquet family as possible and were not designed for public consumption; they were the raw materials of an investigation from which the criminal case against them would be built. This documentation gives us, in contrast to the press, detailed information about the Fiquet couple—their family, habits, and behaviors—and the lives of the other actors in the story. The focus of this chapter will be on the layers of narrative contained in the dossier, in the form of witness statements, interrogations, letters, and other miscellaneous items. Much of this informative material was suppressed in later iterations of the case, but it offers evidence to support a psychodynamic explanation for Fiquet's behavior as rooted in a pathological compulsion to repeat.

The first piece of written evidence in the investigation file was a note signed by two police officers summarizing the initial questioning of two key witnesses that occurred in the hours after Henriette's body was discovered. The first witness, a man named Gallimard, was a thirty-one-year-old rope maker whose workshop was situated on the left bank of the canal, some three hundred meters (330 yards) from the place where Henriette was found. He stated that he had seen a woman whose clothes "seemed to be brown in color."[13] By the time Gallimard's official statement was taken, a week later on 6 July 1882 and following a flurry of press speculation, his recollection had shifted: "She was dressed in black, of medium height. . . . She was wearing some kind of black hat."[14] A brown dress would have made Fiquet resemble any ordinary woman of her class, but the image of a woman in black connoted danger and would have distinguished her symbolically from the image of an ordinary, honest, and virtuous working woman.

The *Côte-d'Or* contrasted this potent image with that of "the little girls in white," who surrounded Henriette's coffin at the funeral procession just days after her body had been found. These girls were the victim's classmates, carrying wreaths of white flowers. One of them was, reportedly, "scarcely able to suppress her sobbing, without doubt Henriette's friend."[15] This emotive emphasis and speculation on what Henriette's loss meant to her community drew a hard moral line between the femme Fiquet and the victim's family. The *Démocratie Bourguignonne* reported the same event without drawing such stark symbolic contrasts between dark and light: "Her little classmates all brought wreaths for her, and this morning, at half past eight, they accompanied her to her final resting place."[16] Nevertheless, the innocence of the victim was still asserted via images of children and funeral flowers and through the contrasting presentation of Fiquet as a suspicious woman. The dead girl's father, Athanäse Barbey, would be cast as an *honnête ouvrier* (a decent, working man), without reproach in the eyes of his employers.

This idea would be reaffirmed in the press coverage of the trial, which eventually took place in the first week of March 1883. In the Parisian press, which picked up the case at the time of the trial, *La Justice* described the Barbey family as "good and honest workers," while *Le Droit populaire* and *Le Figaro* called them "good workers of the city." This strategy was commonly adopted in press reporting of such crimes and had been rehearsed in the case of the Troppmann affair (1869), when a migrant worker from Alsace murdered a whole family, apparently for financial gain. The victims in this earlier case were depicted as decent, hardworking folk, and their killer, Jean-Baptiste Troppmann, as a deranged and motiveless maniac.[17] The reality was murkier, and, as we shall see in the interlude following chapter 4, there was less clear moral water between victim and assailant than the press suggested.

Fiquet's refusal, shortly after her arrest, to look at Henriette's dead body was interpreted by journalists as an indication of callous heartlessness.[18] Yet, her reaction was ambiguous and might equally suggest remorse or confusion because she could not explain, even to herself, what had driven her to kill the child. The coverage of the case fitted Lisa Downing's observation that "the 'ordinary person' . . . must retroactively *become* the extraordinary monster described in the press during the course of a murder hunt."[19] In reality, many elements of Marie-Françoise Fiquet's life and behavior were akin to those around her; she shared the desires and concerns of many of her neighbors and coworkers—indeed, her ordinariness was what made the crime so shocking.

Pierre Fiquet's eventual acquittal and sympathetic treatment by the jury were prefigured by the leniency the press extended to him in July 1882. As the *Catholique* argued, though the femme Fiquet had "named her husband as her accomplice," few were convinced by this "denunciation," since he "passes for an honest worker, whose behavior has been without reproach until now."[20] Pierre Fiquet was presented as being in thrall to his wife's machinations, the pawn to her black queen, an image we shall return to later in this analysis.

In the *dossier de procédure*, numerous minor charges against Pierre Fiquet for petty theft and dishonesty were recorded, so he was not exactly the paragon of decent, working-class virtue presented by the press. Nonetheless, while Fiquet's crime was "committed savagely" and with "chilling premeditation," her husband was immediately exonerated. As the *Côte-d'Or* announced within days of his arrest, "All that we can say is that [Pierre] Fiquet . . . is not the principal actor in this case."[21] We know from comparable cases that female accomplices and onlookers have often been judged as harshly in the court of public opinion as the men who were the primary attackers in each case.[22] It is therefore difficult to believe that, had the roles been reversed, Marie-Françoise Fiquet would have been offered the lenient treatment her husband received.

In contrast to these press reports, from the archive material we gain an extraordinary, layered portrait of the perpetrator—as well as of her victim and of the ordinary people of Dijon—that is humanizing and direct but inconclusive, sometimes incoherent, and self-contradicting. There was also an important power dynamic at play in these interactions, which is reflected in the surviving documentation. The lines of questioning and decisions about whom to interrogate were controlled by the investigating magistrate, and the approach taken depended on the status and existing reputation of the interviewee.

There is a temptation, as Philippe Lejeune has observed, to view these power dynamics in terms of Foucault's conceptualization of power and resistance and to frame a violent crime as "a symbolic protest against the injustices that crush an individual or his social group."[23] Via such a lens we might view Fiquet's actions as having a wider social meaning and offering a commentary on the times in which she lived. This interpretation makes sense, especially if we view her destructive behavior as rooted in trauma and perversion—an argument that I shall develop in chapter 3. However, such neat solutions rarely explain all the elements of a story. The interrogations of Marie-Françoise Fiquet reveal, conversely, the strangeness of the self to the self and the dark places of human motivation. The remainder of this chapter will focus on the information that emerged through the questioning of the main actors in the story during the months following the crime.

Henriette's father, Athanäse Barbey, was called in for questioning on 30 June, the day his daughter's body was discovered. Barbey was a cobbler who, according to this first statement, lived at number 48 rue Berbisey, in central Dijon—a ten-minute walk from the Fiquet family home in rue Musette:

My daughter Henriette was born on 4 December 1876. I have two other younger children. I live with my mother-in-law and my sister-in-law who is twelve or thirteen years old. My daughter Henriette had been going to the infant school for about a year, we always used to let her go alone because she would often meet her school friends. She was in the habit of coming home with her aunt who went to the primary school. . . . Yesterday, on Thursday, Henriette went to school as usual, at eleven o'clock it seems she left as usual with the little Barreau girl, but seeing she had not come back home at the normal time, I went to ask the little Barreau girl why my daughter had not come home. . . . This morning they brought me my child's body, that they had just removed from the canal. I noticed that she didn't have her earrings; they were little [*illeg.*] with blue [*illeg.*] that had cost me six francs. I do not know if my daughter died the victim of an act of vengeance, but my wife and I do not have any enemies. I cannot explain to myself why someone took this child to kill her.[24]

The investigation set out to discover the explanation that eluded Mr. Barbey.

Marie-Françoise Fiquet, who was thirty-one at the time of her arrest, had been born in May 1851 in La Résie-Saint-Martin, a small rural commune in the Haute-Saône Department, some fifty kilometers (thirty-two miles) east of Dijon. Fiquet's father, Jean-Baptiste Rémond, had served in the French army—the family had lived abroad during his career, as a brief remark in the press reporting on the trial in 1883 noted that she had been "raised beneath the African sun." At the time of her arrest, she stood 1.49 meters (4'11") tall, with black hair and eyebrows, brown eyes, a pronounced brow line, an "ordinary nose, medium-sized mouth, round chin, oval face, sallow complexion." The femme Fiquet was *sans profession*—that is, a casual worker without regular employment. Her husband, Pierre, was a native of Noironte, another small rural village further east of Dijon, near the large town of Besançon. Born in November 1853, he was some eighteen months younger than his wife and was described as a *journalier*—an unskilled, casual worker. According to his physical description, he was 1.64 meters (5'5") tall with brown hair and eyebrows, "blond beard, broad forehead, light brown eyes, long nose, medium-sized mouth, round chin, oval face, ruddy complexion."[25]

The French Third Republic penal code categorized felonies against the person in specific ways, which is relevant here because of the various accusations made against the Fiquet couple, beyond killing Henriette. They were accused of "assassinat," the capital crime of murder with premeditation. "Meurtre" in French was reserved for murder committed without premeditation but with clear intent to kill. Special categories also existed for parricide, the killing of a parent or guardian, and poisoning. These crimes were punished with great severity because they were considered cowardly, unnatural, and notoriously difficult to prove. Although the Fiquets were accused of premeditated murder, child killing was not, according to this hierarchy, the very worst crime they could have committed. The accusations of poisoning that would later be levied against the femme Fiquet were as significant as the crime for which she was finally convicted.[26]

The police's first witness, Gallimard, the rope maker who resided near the canal port, stated that at around 10:15 p.m. he saw a woman, apparently dressed in black, walking with a child near to the spot where Henriette's body was discovered. Gallimard noticed it was very late for a woman to be walking to the Pont de Larrey at that time and that she had acted suspiciously: "This woman was holding by her right hand a little girl who she pulled towards her upon seeing me."[27] When Gallimard was placed in "confrontation" with the femme Fiquet, he was not positively able to identify her, but he affirmed that he had seen a woman of her height and that Henriette had been wearing light-colored tights.[28] Another witness, Edmé Michel, a thirty-two-year-old customs officer whose post was situated adjacent to the bridge, stated that he saw a man and a woman walking along the canal with a child at around 10:30 p.m.[29]

To the examining magistrate, Alfred Loiseau, it became quickly apparent that the femme Fiquet was responsible for the death of Henriette Barbey. But his interrogations also gradually drew out details of her everyday life experiences, including poverty, addiction, and physical struggles. Fiquet's early adult life had begun with the experience, all too common for poor, young women, of being almost perpetually in a state of pregnancy, child-birth, child-rearing, and child loss. But the details of these losses would only emerge as the investigation progressed. As we shall see, the pieces of the puzzle that was Marie-Françoise Fiquet's life would not come together in strict chronological order.

This is not surprising because, as Ann-Louise Shapiro has suggested, the stories that emerge from judicial dossiers are "stories-in-tension."[30] Crime narratives are invariably composed of competing versions of the same story, from cultural myths to official reports to the alternative and oppositional stories offered by defendants:

> It was not uncommon for women who committed violent acts during this period to immediately turn themselves in to the local police commissioner. At this initial interrogation, it is especially striking that these women tended *not* to discuss the crime itself, but rather to rehearse a litany of longstanding grievances captured in a selected sequence of events that were meant to account for the crime in some much broader sense than the immediate provocation. By means of these narratives, women identified the particular moments that, in their minds, gave coherence and legitimacy to their lives, even when the logic of the story was quite different from the versions that were ultimately constructed through the judicial process.[31]

We shall see that the femme Fiquet, through these early interrogations, offered her own account of her life and actions that was in tension with the simplified narrative of her as a denatured killer.

Fiquet's reactions to the judge's questions asked in the first few interrogations following her arrest, which took place from 30 June to 10 November

1882, alternated between denial, amnesia, blame, silence, and—finally—a confession, which she later retracted.[32] In the first interrogation, conducted on 30 June 1882, the day Henriette's body was found, the investigating magistrate confronted Fiquet directly with the evidence the investigators gained from the girl who had seen her at the school gates, fourteen-year-old Louise Coquereaux: "Did you not take the little girl named Henriette Barbey by the hand telling her, come to my house, your mummy is waiting for you there?" Fiquet replied, "It is not true."[33] She was then placed in confrontation with Coquereaux, who again insisted that Fiquet was the woman she had seen talking to Henriette at the school gates. The accused woman again denied everything and suggested that Coquereaux was motivated by a grudge, following a petty argument at the tobacco factory where they had both worked. How long Fiquet was employed there is unknown, but, as we learn from several key documents in the dossier, she suddenly quit her job at the factory just days before Henriette was found dead. This, she would later explain, was because her driving ambition had been to work as a midwife.

Fiquet was then asked about her movements on the day before Henriette's body was found. She explained to Loiseau that she had gone home to eat lunch with her daughter, Louise, at midday: "My husband, who had been in hospital, returned home at midday. A moment later my daughter left to go back to the tobacco factory. My husband and I went downstairs to the Tisserands' restaurant, they were in front of their door. We stayed there about ten minutes, from there my husband and I went to the cemetery, we stayed there at least two hours, from two o'clock to four o'clock, we chatted to all the gravediggers, then we came home, and I prepared supper."

The significance of the Fiquet couple's mysterious visits to the cemetery and the graves of two infants there was not yet evident to the investigating magistrate. However, as would later transpire, the dead children were apparently the Fiquets' twin babies, who had died in 1881. A further detail, which would be significant, was revealed when Loiseau asked, "Did you know that your husband was meant to leave hospital today?" Fiquet replied, "Yes, they had told me that at the hospital."[34] In the third interrogation, the femme Fiquet finally admitted that she had been involved in Henriette's abduction and had brought the child back to their apartment. But she insisted that it was her husband who had killed Henriette out of revenge. According to the femme Fiquet, her husband had accused her of having an affair with the victim's father, Athanäse Barbey.

> He [Pierre Fiquet] reproached me for having had relations with Barbey, whom I do not know. I assured him that I had never had relations with

him. . . . He told me that Barbey had a little girl who went to the school, that he would take her at the school exit and that he would take her home to her parents. On Thursday 29 June . . . I went down the rue St Philibert to go and meet my husband who was meant to be leaving hospital. . . . He's the one who showed me the little Barbey girl, he told me to take her home to our house. The little girl followed me and the three of us went back to our house.[35]

The story about the affair was denied by all concerned, including Henriette's father, and Pierre Fiquet initially also denied all knowledge of Henriette's presence in his home on 29 June.[36] His wife then claimed she had been acting in a drug haze and had no clear recollection of what had happened: "I took too much chloroform that day, I no longer remember what was said."[37]

In the seventh interrogation, Loiseau asked, "You told me when you accused your husband . . . that he had pushed the little girl in the water, that she had not cried. Is it not you who did that and not your husband?" The femme Fiquet replied, "I don't remember."[38] In the eighth interrogation, she finally confessed both to bringing the child back to her apartment and to having pushed her into the canal: "When Fiquet had gone to bed, I woke the child, she did not cry and said nothing to me. . . . I don't know how I pushed her towards the water, I don't remember having met any other people apart from two men working at the customs (octroi) gate, in front of the Lamy headquarters. . . . I did not ask the little girl who she was or where she lived."[39] In the next interrogation, Fiquet was asked why she had sought to implicate her husband. "I don't know what I did to involve him in this affair," she replied. "I acknowledge that he has nothing to do with it."[40] This was the only time the woman admitted that she had killed Henriette, that she had acted alone, and that the girl was alive when she had left her apartment with her.

Fiquet quickly retracted her confession, and, in her last depositions, she again blamed her husband. "I have searched my mind and now I am convinced that it is not me who drowned the little girl," she declared.[41] She told her story in a dissociative way, as though from a distance, evoking the chilling image of watching her husband nonchalantly drown the child: "Fiquet told me that he held the little girl's head in the water with his umbrella."[42] It later emerged that Pierre Fiquet had indeed seen more than he had initially claimed, but he strenuously denied the accusation of murder.

The first police interrogation of Pierre Fiquet took place on 1 July in the section house at the railroad crossing in the hamlet of Pichanges, in the commune of Marsannay-le-Bois, twenty-eight kilometers (seventeen miles) north of Dijon. In his statement Pierre Fiquet said he had gone there to stay with his brother; he stated his profession as a candlemaker and gave an account of his movements on 29 June. Prior to the murder, he said, he had been in hospital in Dijon for three weeks recovering from a stomach illness. He had left hospital on Thursday, 29 June and gone directly home, ate lunch with his wife, then went to see Zimmerman the candlemaker at the canal port to seek work for the following week.

Then, reported Mr. Fiquet, "I went home around two o'clock, without stopping anywhere. Around three o'clock, I went with my wife to the cemetery. We planted a few flowers on our children's grave. I stayed there until about half past five. I even saw a burial while I was there. I went home directly with my wife without stopping and I did not go out again. I did not receive a visit from anyone. I left Dijon on Friday morning on foot, around six o'clock."[43] Mr. Fiquet's daughter had left at dawn to go to work at the factory. He did not have enough money to buy a train ticket, so he had walked all the way to his brother's house and arrived in the evening. It would have been unclear to investigators what Pierre Fiquet meant by his "children's grave," but this detail would later prove a key element to Marie-Françoise Fiquet's strange story.

Mr. Fiquet's second interrogation took place back in Dijon on 2 July. He was asked again about his movements and to specify whom he had seen. He maintained that he had not seen a child at his home apart from his daughter, Louise, who had come home for lunch. Loiseau then placed Pierre Fiquet, at this point named in procedural documents as his wife's co-accused, l'inculpé, in a confrontation with his daughter. Thirteen-year-old Louise Fiquet asserted, "I did not see my father when I came back from the factory, he did not have lunch with my mother, the little girl and me. I even asked my mother if he would come home soon. She replied that he would probably come home later that day."[44] Louise's testimony suggested that Pierre Fiquet was lying about the timings of his movements that day, perhaps repeating a script given to him by his wife.

Fiquet was then placed in confrontation with her husband, which was recorded in the same interrogation report. She accused her husband directly: "It's you who carried the little girl, wrapped in a shawl, and pushed her with an umbrella. That's what he told me in the morning."[45] Following this allegation, the examining magistrate asked Mr. Fiquet how he and his wife had met. "I left military service in June 1875. I had a certificate for good behavior, and I went home to my parents. . . . My father worked at the mill owned by Mr. Grébille. Marie Raymond [sic] lived with my father and mother, she had moved with them from Vitreux. She had her child [Louise] with her. She also worked at Mr. Grébille's mill. I did not have relations with her at that time."

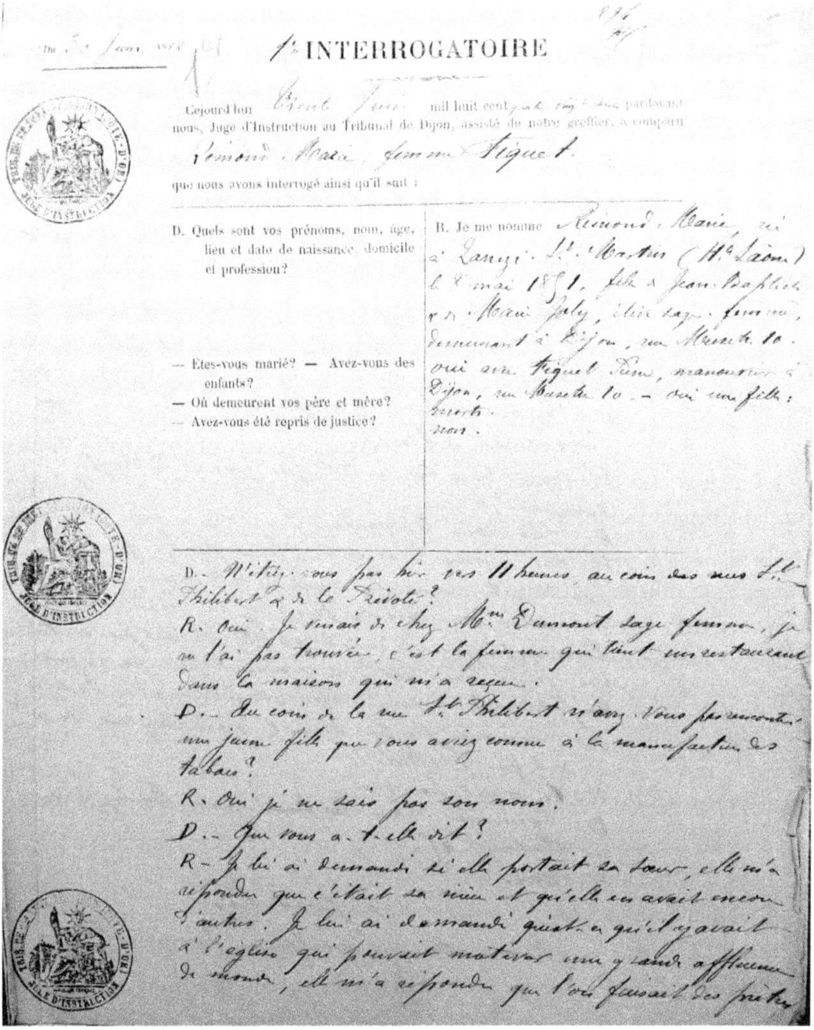
Du 30 Juin 1883

1er INTERROGATOIRE

Cejourd'hui trente Juin mil huit cent quatre vingt trois par devant nous, Juge d'Instruction au Tribunal de Dijon, assisté de notre greffier, a comparu Rémond Marie femme Fiquet

que nous avons interrogé ainsi qu'il suit :

D. Quels sont vos prénoms, nom, âge, lieu et date de naissance, domicile et profession?

R. Je me nomme Rémond, Marie, née à Lanty St Martin (Hte Saône) le 8 mai 1851, fille de Jean-Baptiste et de Marie Joly, élève sage-femme, demeurant à Dijon, rue Musette 10.

— Etes-vous marié? — Avez-vous des enfants?
— Où demeurent vos père et mère?
— Avez-vous été repris de justice?

oui avec Fiquet Pierre, manouvrier à Dijon, rue Musette 10. — oui une fille; morts. non.

D.— N'étiez-vous pas hier vers 11 heures au coin des rues St Philibert et de la Prévôté?

R. Oui je venais de chez Mme Dumont sage femme, je ne l'ai pas trouvée, c'est la femme qui tient un restaurant dans la maison qui m'a reçue.

D.— Au coin de la rue St Philibert n'avez-vous pas rencontré une jeune fille que vous aviez connue à la manufacture des tabacs?

R. Oui je ne sais pas son nom.

D.— Que vous a-t-elle dit?

R.— Je lui ai demandé si elle portait sa sœur, elle m'a répondu que c'était sa nièce et qu'elle en avait encore d'autres. Je lui ai demandé ce qu'il y avait à l'église qui pouvait motiver une grande affluence de monde, elle m'a répondu que l'on faisait des prières

FIGURE 2. First interrogation of Marie-Françoise Fiquet, 30 June 1883. Courtesy of the Archives Départementales de la Côte-d'Or in Dijon.

In 1877, he and Marie-Françoise Rémond, as she was called then, moved to Épinal, where they stayed for three years, during which time they married. He was Catholic, and she was Protestant, but he had wanted a Catholic wedding. He added, "I even legally recognized her child, who was not mine."[46]

The marriage would later be described as loveless by numerous witnesses and even by the femme Fiquet herself during police interrogations. Her decision to marry Pierre Fiquet was a pragmatic one, and in many respects, it was a self-protective move. Unmarried poor women who were either pregnant or alone with children were among the most vulnerable people in society, and having the security of a man's wage to support the family could be the difference between surviving and dying. The Napoleonic Code also expressly forbid women from legally pursuing the father of a child.[47] In addition to these practical concerns, Pierre loved his adopted daughter, Louise, and raised her as his own.

Both parents displayed some religious devotion and saw to the baptism and religious instruction of their only daughter. Fiquet was adept at convincing people to give her money and even persuaded a priest to fund a visit to the restorative waters at Plombières for her.[48] Their interest in the two religious traditions was interpreted as cynical maneuvering by the investigation. However, the letters and statements, and the couple's habit of ritually visiting graveyards, suggest an attraction to spiritual matters that went beyond simple self-interest. This complicates the press narrative of the femme Fiquet as a reckless and amoral woman. She embodied certain traits of both the model Christian woman, who took her daughter's religious education seriously, and the scandalous woman whose personal morality and sexual licentiousness conflicted with the moral code she apparently endorsed.[49]

The family had moved to Dijon in July 1880, Pierre Fiquet explained, "because my wife wanted to learn to be a midwife. Wherever we lived my wife spent time in hospitals." The questioning continued. In February 1881, he had traveled to Moissey, a village in the Jura mountains, to stay with his parents, and he had taken Louise with him. During this time, he claimed, his wife had stayed in Dijon to take midwifery classes, and he had received a letter from her claiming that she had given birth to twins. He rushed home to find his wife alone, and she told him the twins had died.

After that time, they regularly visited the cemetery where he believed the babies were buried. "I then went to work as an operator at the railway shunting yard, up until the time I fell ill. My wife wanted to stop me going to hospital because she thought I could recover just as well at home."[50] These clues in Pierre Fiquet's story were the first indications of his wife's disordered behavior. It would later be revealed that she had never given birth to twins, that she had been ejected from midwifery classes, and that she had actively prevented her seriously ill husband from accessing hospital care. Her quietly destructive behavior and morbid fascination with death and babies would later prove important clues to her motivations.

In the fifth interrogation, which took place on 6 July, Pierre Fiquet told the investigators that on the day he had returned home from hospital, he had gone to buy a pair of trousers in the rue Berbisey for four francs, with money his father had sent to help him buy necessities, and then he went home. He continued to claim that he had never seen Henriette. But, after almost a month of interrogations, at the end of July 1882, Pierre Fiquet wrote a letter to the examining magistrate in which he changed his story, stating he had arrived home at one o'clock in the afternoon on the 29 June to find his wife in the bedroom and the little Barbey girl lying on the bed. Called in to explain himself, Mr. Fiquet stated, "It's true, I didn't notice if the child was alive or dead. When I came back from Zimmerman's by the canal, the little girl was no longer in my wife's bedroom, I didn't see her, but my wife told me that she was dead. I didn't see her either when we came back from the cemetery. I only saw her again at ten o'clock when my wife carried her away."

The magistrate demanded, "Is it not you who took the child's comb and earrings?" "I did not touch the child," Pierre Fiquet replied. Loiseau continued, "Why did you not alert the authorities about what happened at your home on the 29 June, since you claim to be innocent?" Mr. Fiquet, in a state of remorse, simply replied, "I was wrong not to do so."[51]

In the tenth interrogation, on 2 August, Pierre Fiquet gave further details of what he had actually seen that day. He told Loiseau that he had returned home in the afternoon to find his wife in a state of panic. A child she had brought home had apparently died after accidentally drinking some morphine solution that she had prepared for herself, since she was a habitual drug user. He described the scene that greeted him:

> When I came home from the hospital the little girl was sleeping on my wife's bed and my wife told me that she was a sick child that she had found in the street. . . . The little girl was in the bedroom next to us, and my wife was crying, and she told me that the little girl was dead. . . . When I came home with my wife around ten o'clock [in the evening], the little girl was on my bed, my wife took her and wrapped her in a shawl, she made it look like a bundle of laundry and she left carrying the child, she said she was going to leave her in a passageway, I don't know where, and that after that she would go to the canal side, that I was to meet her there. That is what I did. I remember meeting a man on the bridge. . . . The officer was at the toll gate. . . . I walked past the ropemakers, the lights were on. I finally found my wife, she was sitting at the edge of the water, the little girl was lying in the water, my wife told me to push her towards the middle, I replied, "Now you have really pulled it off, this has nothing to do with me." We returned taking the Gemeaux path, my wife walking ahead. . . . When we got home I went to bed and I did not ask my wife for any kind of explanation. I only learnt the details of the affair after my arrest.[52]

Admitting he was wrong not to raise the alarm when he found the girl, Pierre Fiquet appeared to express remorse for his lack of action and conceded that he should have told the truth earlier: "I really should have said it." His wife's behavior and responses, however, revealed her to be a calculating and disturbed personality who was capable of violence. As we know already, the eyewitnesses Gallimard and Michel claimed to have seen the child alive late in the evening. Therefore, in asserting to her husband that the little girl was already dead, earlier in the day, the femme Fiquet seemed to have been rehearsing the idea of killing Henriette even as she lay asleep, possibly drugged. It also indicates that even at this stage, her husband's account was still not entirely truthful.

In the eleventh interrogation of Pierre Fiquet, on 19 October 1882, Loiseau pursued a line of questioning about the history of the Fiquet family, including where they had met and how they had lived. Mr. Fiquet noted that the family had moved around frequently to find work and that his wife preferred staying in places where she could easily access a doctor. A type of "medical nomadism," typical of factitious disorders, is commonly noted in case histories in the medical literature.[53] Mr. Fiquet added detail to his earlier account, telling Loiseau that he had come home only to find his wife in tears: "I offered to carry the child to the police station, she didn't want me to." But he denied carrying the child to the canal, as his wife had accused him of doing: "I have told the honest truth," he said, and repeated his regret that he had not confessed what he had seen earlier in proceedings.

As I discovered when retracing their steps along the route in Dijon, from the Fiquets' home at 10 rue Musette to the Pont de Larrey and to the spot where Henriette was found, the journey is a brisk thirty-minute walk. It would have been impossible for a chronically drug-addicted, sick, emaciated woman in narcotic withdrawal to carry a five-year-old child that distance, alive or dead. This was a point Marie-Françoise Fiquet herself made in a letter to the investigating magistrate: "I could not have carried her from one room to the other," she claimed, suggesting either that her husband must have carried the child some of the way or that Henriette was alive and walked with them to the canal.[54]

During the twelfth interrogation, on 10 November, the investigators continued to put pressure on Pierre Fiquet as a possible accomplice to the crime. According to him, when the child was in the water, his wife said to him, "Push her out into the water a bit, the boats will carry her away. I replied to her that it had nothing to do with me. I had an umbrella with me the whole time and my wife wanted me to push the little girl with that umbrella. . . . I was wrong not to tell the truth the day of my arrest."

The letters written by the Fiquet couple and retained in the case dossier reveal an intellectual gulf between husband and wife. Pierre's letters are illegible and only semiliterate, while his wife's, despite her limited education, are relatively well composed and detailed. Mr. Fiquet's intellectual limitations would be observed repeatedly through the case proceedings by investigators, doctors, and reporters, and were not only due to a lack of formal education. Despite his apparently low intelligence, Pierre Fiquet demonstrated empathy and kindness, and despite his inaction, he exhibited a clear moral sense of right and wrong when faced with the dilemma of what to do with the abducted child. His wife seemed to be in the grip of a different sort of urge entirely.

Throughout the interviews, it never became entirely clear whether Henriette was dead, drugged with morphine, or alive and well when she left the Fiquets' apartment. It is possible that she was temporarily drugged earlier in the day, if the story about the morphine solution is to be believed, but later drowned when she was placed in the water. The autopsy and witness reports suggested that the child was alive and awake when she reached the canal. Dr. Deroye, who carried out an initial examination of the child's body, reported the cause of death as drowning following submersion in water less than twelve hours previously, finding evidence of "the aspiration of liquid and its rejection by coughing." Deroye also found that the child's stomach was distended, filled with liquid and partially digested pieces of fruit, meaning that Henriette had eaten the food given to her by the femme Fiquet. The chemical analysis of the stomach contents was inconclusive, finding no trace either of morphine or arsenic, although the investigators could not rule out the presence of toxins because the stomach was full of water.[55]

Marie-Françoise Fiquet's life as a habitual morphine user briefly proved an important feature of her case, and the *dossier de procédure* gives direct insights into this element of her existence. Fiquet reported that she had been using morphine for two years, following treatment for a spinal problem. Her daughter said she was sent to the pharmacist each day to fetch either a gram or half a gram of morphine for her mother, who could access the drug without charge through city funds because the family was classed as indigent.[56] The dossier contains medical bills from local pharmacists detailing the femme Fiquet's consumption over a period of several months. For example, according to one note from the pharmacist A. Raynaud, 18 rue Chaudronnerie, for "medicines supplied to Madame Fiquet, 10 rue Musette" from August to December 1881, she was obtaining one gram of chloralhydrate of morphine twice per month—and this was only one of her suppliers.

If Fiquet was taking even half a gram of morphine per day, as suggested by her daughter, this was a relatively high dose. If she had not been able to take morphine in the habitual way via injection, she would likely have been

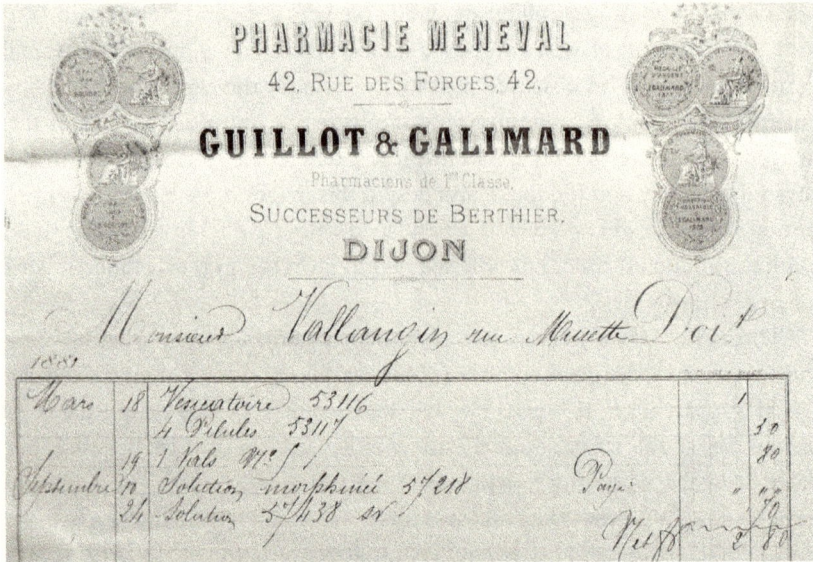

FIGURE 3A. Morphine prescription and medical supplies, 1881. Courtesy of the Archives Départementales de la Côte-d'Or in Dijon.

experiencing withdrawal symptoms.[57] Crucially, Fiquet stated that when her arms were too scarred or when her syringes had broken, she was in the habit of drinking morphine in a sugar solution; this was why she had the liquid medicine in her home when Henriette was there. In his statement to police, a silversmith named Vincent Schettine confirmed that the femme Fiquet had brought her syringe to him for repair three days before Henriette's death and had returned to collect it on 29 June, declaring she had "overwhelming need" of the instrument, but he had not yet had time to fix it.[58] This suggests Fiquet's usual drug routine had been interrupted, and she was therefore under stress on the day of Henriette's abduction. Her claim to have taken substitutes like chloroform and the sugared morphine solution is therefore convincing, but her state remained destabilized. Finally, had Henriette ingested any of the morphine solution, she would have been at least sedated, if not in mortal danger.

Despite the evidence that Fiquet was in withdrawal at the time of Henriette's death, this would not have excused her actions in the eyes of the law. This is because, as Sara Black has demonstrated in her detailed research on the question of legal medicine and criminal responsibility in late nineteenth-century France, morphine withdrawal was only considered an excuse for theft of money or goods to obtain the addictive drug. Black found that experts did not consider the effects of morphine itself (or morphine with-

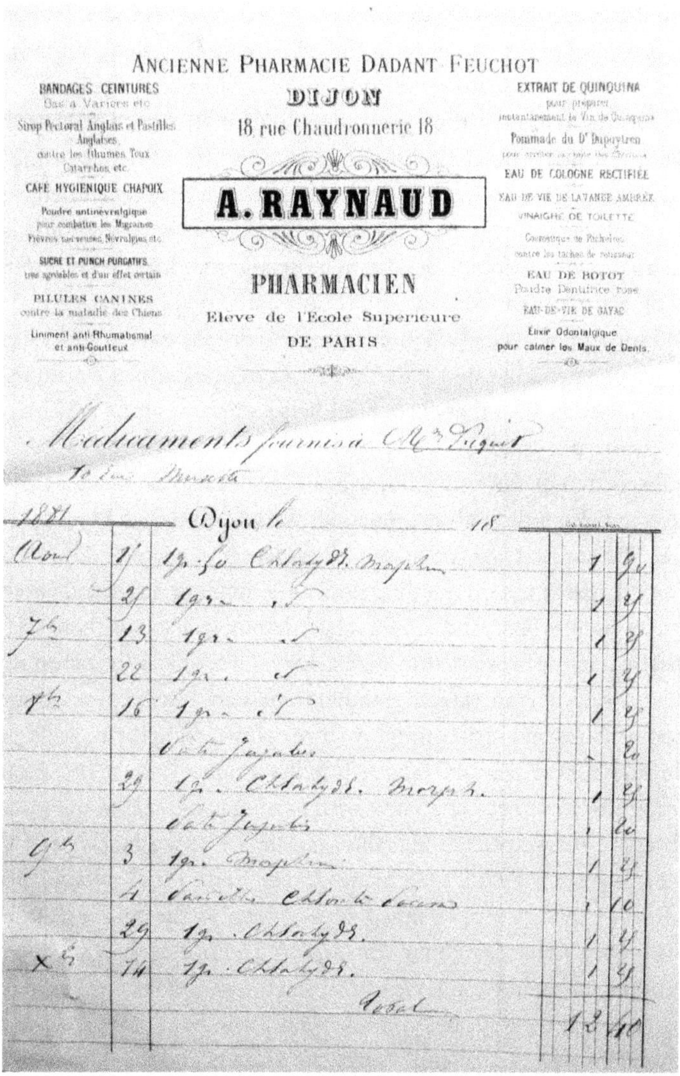
ANCIENNE PHARMACIE DADANT FEUCHOT

DIJON

18 rue Chaudronnerie 18

A. RAYNAUD

PHARMACIEN

Elève de l'Ecole Superieure

DE PARIS

BANDAGES CEINTURES

Bas a Varices etc

Sirop Pectoral Anglais et Pastilles Anglaises contre les Rhumes Toux Catarrhes etc.

CAFÉ HYGIENIQUE CHAPOIX

Poudre antinévralgique pour combattre les Migraines

SUCRE ET PUNCH PURGATIFS

PILULES CANINES

contre la maladie des Chiens

Liniment anti Rhumatismal et anti-Goutteux

EXTRAIT DE QUINQUINA

Pommade du Dr Dupuytren

EAU DE COLOGNE RECTIFIÉE

EAU DE VIE DE LAVANDE AMBRÉE

VINAIGRE DE TOILETTE

EAU DE BOTOT

Poudre Dentifrice rose

EAU-DE-VIE DE GAYAC

Elixir Odontalgique pour calmer les Maux de Dents.

FIGURE 3B. Morphine prescription and medical supplies, 1881. Courtesy of the Archives Départementales de la Côte-d'Or in Dijon.

drawal) sufficient to alter a person's character and *cause* someone to commit a violent crime: "Addicted defendants claimed that morphine produced a state of temporary insanity. However, medical-legal experts emphasized the more complex regulatory influence of morphine over the addicted body—specifically, morphine's capacity to relieve pain, soothe anxiety, and stave off withdrawal symptoms of its own making."[59] Prosecutors would therefore have argued against Fiquet's claim to have been negatively affected by morphine on the grounds that the drug was believed to pacify users. It apparently did not drive people to violence in the same way that alcohol often could. In Fiquet's case, it made no sense to claim that morphine made her commit murder. On the contrary, the experts would ultimately decide that she was responsible for her actions *because* she was under the influence of morphine rather than disturbed by it, as the femme Fiquet (at times) claimed.

As we shall see in chapter 4, the examining doctors believed Fiquet's claim to inject a gram of morphine per day to be exaggerated. However, contemporary medical treatises and fictional accounts based on observations of addicts recorded morphine users (whether men or women) injecting between one and two grams per day—and sometimes more: for example, Dr. Louis Raoul Régnier claimed in 1890 that chronic addicts sometimes took as much as two to three grams per day.[60]

The inspection of the family home at 10 rue Musette soon after the Fiquets were arrested also indicated that narcotics were central to the femme Fiquet's daily life. The account written by the investigating magistrate described a tiny two-roomed apartment on the third floor of a building that stood above a restaurant run by the Tisserand family. The building still stands there today, and rue Musette is in the heart of commercial Dijon; it is one of the oldest streets in the city, and today it is an attractive, rather upmarket, busy pedestrian street full of boutique shops and luxury grocery stores, showcasing the region's prosperity.[61] Throughout the year, and especially in the warmer months, the shop fronts open out onto the streets, animated with passing trade due to the location of the impressive marketplace, the Halles du Marché, just a block away. Despite its modernization, the little road retains the feel of a medieval street, with its cobbled paving and nearby winding streets, such as the rue des Forges. The narrow bustling streets lead up to the imposing edifice of the church of Notre Dame and its square, forming one of the neighborhood's central focal points.

It has been a gentrified area for many years now, but in 1882 it was a district that housed working-class families like the Fiquets and the Barbeys who had come to Dijon to take advantage of employment opportunities created by industrialization and the development of the railways. The wholesalers with their large, accessible premises were situated at the edge of the city, near the canal for the receipt of goods. Smaller shops and markets serving the needs of workers and residents were concentrated in the city center. Dijon would not open its first major department store, "La Ménagère," which occupied an entire block of the main street, the rue de la Liberté, until five years later in 1887.[62] Paris already had three major stores, including "Le Bon Marché," and was entering its shopping heyday. The examining magistrate's notes in the dossier described the apartment as a scene of destitution and neglect

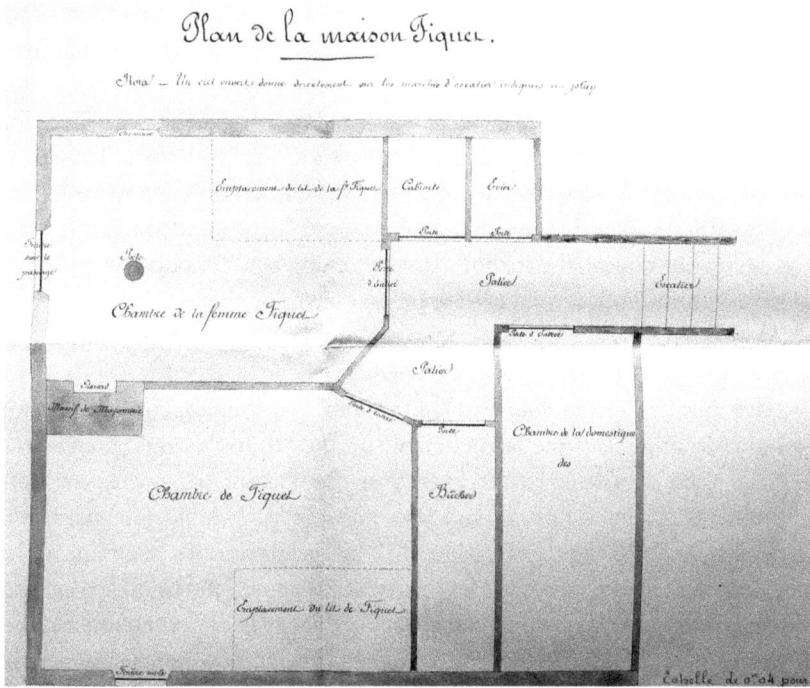

FIGURE 4. Interior plan of the Fiquet family apartment at 10 rue Musette. Courtesy of the Archives Départementales de la Côte-d'Or in Dijon.

explicitly linked to Fiquet's drug dependency: "The furniture consists of a bed, in both bedrooms, which are in a terrible state. Little or no bedlinen. In all corners of the bedrooms there are all kinds of rags. Old books, empty bottles, coming from all kinds of pharmacies. . . . In the husband's bedroom on a little table several old medical textbooks that Fiquet had bought on 27 June. The Fiquet girl gives us a box in which we find bottles containing phials of different pharmaceutical products."[63]

The chemist appointed by the investigation, Philippe-Gustave Héberd, analyzed the contents of the numerous containers taken from the Fiquet home and found chloroform, ether, several opium-based products, orange-flower water, distilled water, sugar syrup, and rose water. His findings matched the details of Fiquet's story, notably her claim that she gave Henriette sugared water to drink and her memory of having taken chloroform. No syringes were found.[64]

The family dynamic that emerged through the Fiquets' statements and letters was that of a dominant mother, a passive and slow-witted father, and a dutiful and devout daughter. Louise Fiquet was questioned by Loiseau as a possible witness, but she was never considered a suspect. Her first statements were taken on 1 and 4 July. In these accounts, Louise confirmed seeing Henriette in the apartment and described her as an extremely shy child, who sat motionless on a chair, said nothing, and refused the carrots she was offered for lunch but agreed to eat a few cherries. Louise returned to work at 12:30 p.m. and came home at 6:20 p.m. She did not see Henriette later in the evening, and when she inquired of the girl's whereabouts, "my mother replied that she had taken her downstairs without anyone seeing her."[65] Louise went to bed at nine o'clock. That she did not see or hear anything that evening, when the child was almost certainly alive and in the tiny family apartment, is puzzling and suggests that Henriette might indeed have been drugged or asleep.

After her parents were arrested, Louise moved to Besançon to live with her grandmother. Despite being fiercely devoted to her mother, Louise was a pious child who realized the gravity of the accusations against her parents. She also trusted Loiseau and wrote him several letters. She was interviewed again on 20 and 26 October 1882 by the authorities in Besançon. In her early statements, given in Dijon, Louise recounted the facts of what she saw at home on the day of Henriette's abduction. In her later statements, she appeared keen to distance herself from the crime and opened her responses with the affirmation, "I am the daughter of the accused, which will not prevent me from telling the truth."[66]

The dossier also contains a letter, written on decorative paper and dated "Dijon, le 31 décembre," from Louise to her mother. The child's use of the formal "vous" form to address her mother and the formulaic but accurate language suggest it was copied from a model letter provided by her teachers to announce Louise's first communion. The letter did not mention Fiquet's crime, arrest, or separation from her daughter. Louise wrote with clear, neat handwriting and expressed gratitude to her mother despite everything that had happened:

> Dear Mama,
>
> On this happy day for me I come to you to express my feelings of affection and gratitude for all your goodness. Each year I am more indebted to you and each year I am more grateful. I can only express this to you by sincere good wishes for your happiness. These are dictated by my heart and God will surely grant them for if he blesses grateful children, he also blesses my good mother. I embrace you tenderly.
>
> Louise Fiquet[67]

A second letter from Louise, addressed to the examining magistrate and contained in the same subfolder, asked him to pass on the news of her first com-

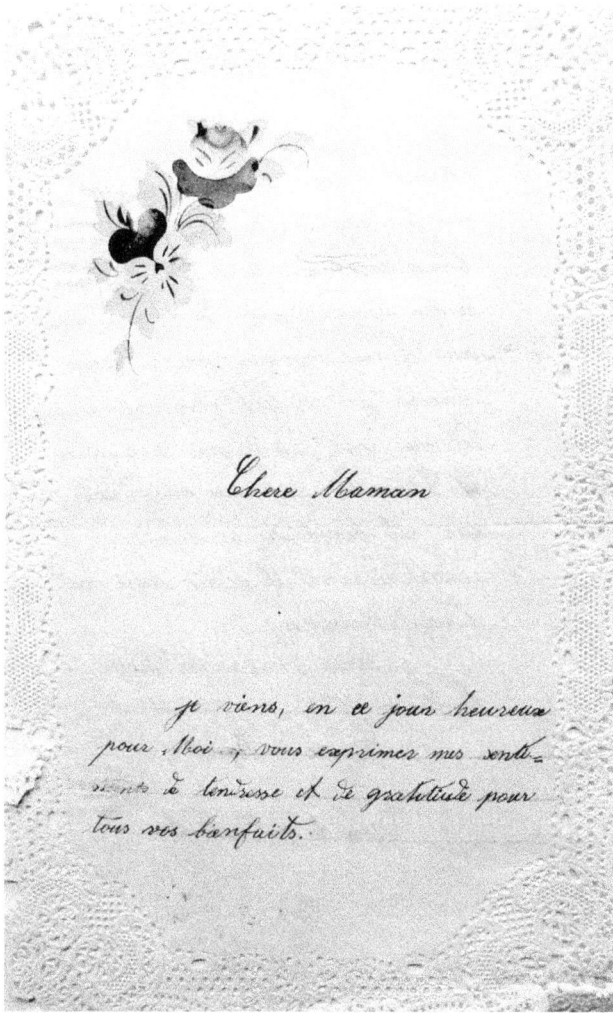

FIGURE 5A.   Letter from Louise Fiquet to her mother, 31 December 1882.
Courtesy of the Archives Départementales de la Côte-d'Or in Dijon.

munion. Both letters were written in the final months of 1882. A pencil note on the second letter records the date of 16 November 1882, and Louise's own writing is comprehensible but full of spelling errors, suggesting she also had only elementary reading and writing skills: "I have set myself the task of letting you know that I am receiving my first communion on Sunday 26 [*illeg.*] that sir would be good enough to let my unfortunate mother know. . . . Thanks to my good parents who [*illeg.*] by the priest and thanks to God, sir, I am obliged to forgive all the bad things and the suffering she has caused me in my life."

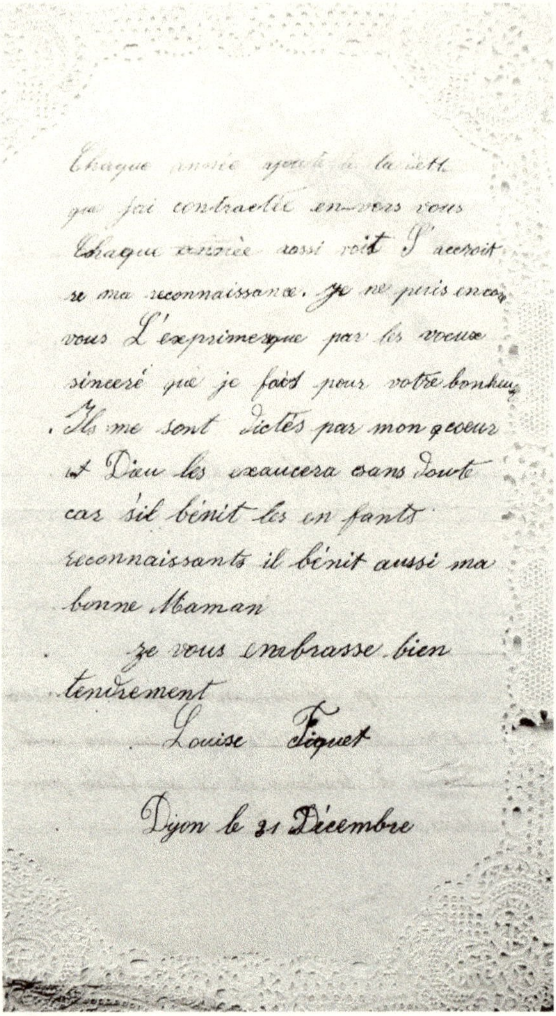

Chaque année ajoute à la dette
que j'ai contractée envers vous
Chaque année aussi voit s'accroître
ma reconnaissance. Je ne puis encore
vous l'exprimer que par les voeux
sincères que je fais pour votre bonheur
Ils me sont dictés par mon coeur
et Dieu les exaucera sans doute
car s'il bénit les enfants
reconnaissants il bénit aussi ma
bonne Maman
je vous embrasse bien
tendrement
Louise Fiquet
Dijon le 31 Décembre

FIGURE 5B. Letter from Louise Fiquet to her mother, 31 December 1882. Courtesy of the Archives Départementales de la Côte-d'Or in Dijon.

The letter expressed Louise's ambivalence: she declared love and gratitude to her parents for bringing her to church and faith, forgiveness for the difficulties they had inflicted on her, and pity for their predicament. At the end of the letter there is a poignant note, as if an afterthought, that reads, "Please say hello to Daddy from his daughter who loves him."[68] Perhaps Louise was under the influence of her religious directors, expressing the sentiment that she should not complain and must forgive her parents for their misdeeds.

We also gain from the dossier a portrait of Henriette, a little girl from a modest family whose early and unnatural death meant that her life is briefly inscribed in the historical record, one of those "ordinary people . . . rarely visited by history" evoked by Arlette Farge.[69] According to her teacher, Henriette was "a reticent child" who "talked very little and rarely played with her classmates. She always seemed very sad. She was not very intelligent. I did not know her parents."[70] Henriette's maternal grandmother, the femme Tissot, testified that Henriette was regularly victimized and terrified of everyone: "The little girl was extremely shy and did not play with other children outside the house. She did not know how to stick up for herself when girls younger than her bullied her."[71] This personality profile suggests she would have been an easy victim for the femme Fiquet.

Henriette's mother, Olympe Tissot, the femme Barbey, confirmed this view, describing her daughter's personality as "rather sad" as well as "very fearful," noting that she was too afraid even to sit on her own father's lap.[72] Henriette's father told the investigators, "The little one was taciturn and not very communicative. . . . She was extremely shy and uncomfortable even with me; she allowed herself to be led astray by little girls much younger than her. She was in fragile health."[73] One person Henriette did seem to trust, if briefly and tragically, was Marie-Françoise Fiquet, who recalled hearing the child say to her husband, "I want to go and be near the lady," to which he replied, "She has gone to get your mummy."[74]

Of course, Fiquet had not gone to fetch Henriette's mother, and these were the last recorded words uttered by a little girl unlucky enough to find herself drawn into a situation much darker and more complex than she could ever have understood. The early stages of the investigation established beyond doubt that Marie-Françoise Fiquet had orchestrated Henriette's abduction, but it was still unclear if Pierre Fiquet was an accomplice or merely a hapless observer. Louise had seen the child, but she was clearly not involved in her mother's plan, and the investigation was satisfied that Henriette's parents also knew nothing about what happened that day. Although the precise details remained unclear, everything circled around the femme Fiquet, and the authorities were sure at least that she had taken Henriette from school for no apparent reason. These early findings meant that the focus of the investigation, beyond establishing Fiquet's movements and contact with Henriette on that fateful day, would shift to consider other elements of the accused woman's life. What kind of person was she? What reputation did she have locally? Was she suspected of other crimes, and had she killed before? And what should the investigation make of her fixation with young children and medical procedures?

CHAPTER 3

The Character Assessment

The investigation into the death of Henriette Barbey assessed the morality of the prime suspect. Marie-Françoise Fiquet's reputation and her capacity for violence became the chief preoccupations of the investigating magistrate. There is a subfolder in the *dossier de procédure* titled "renseignements de moralité" ("information on morality") that takes its reader back chronologically into Marie-Françoise Fiquet's past lives. It contains evidence suggesting that Henriette's death was not a random or arbitrary act but rather the culmination of a sequence of disturbing events. We learn these details only through the testimonies of others and not through Fiquet's own confessions.

The collection of this body of evidence relating to the femme Fiquet's character took place between early July 1882 and November 1882, before the first presentation of the case in the assizes court. James M. Donovan's research on nineteenth- and twentieth-century criminal justice in France is instructive on the type of evidence that was gathered and presented. Donovan has further shown that juries often refused to convict alleged murderers for fear of excessively harsh punishment:

> Such verdicts were facilitated by the nature of trials in the *cours d'assises*, which appear to have often allowed jurors to decide in accordance with their personal sentiments. Much of this bias was due to the fact that

juries often judged on the basis of the accused person's character; the trials were of personalities as much as they were of crimes. This was because of the ways in which evidence was presented, evidence that also appealed more to the emotions than to the reason of jurors. The *cours d'assises* were set up by Napoleon's Code of Criminal Procedure (*Code d'instruction criminelle*) in 1808 to try *crimes* (felonies). They were the only courts in France to use juries. There was one in each *départe-ment*. It was presided over by a *président* (chief justice) and two junior colleagues . . . who voted with the *président* to determine the penalty. Questions of guilt or innocence were decided by twelve jurors. Trial proceedings in the *cours d'assises* were theatrical in nature, and this, along with the active questioning of defendants and witnesses by the *président*, the lack of rules of evidence, and the requirement that jurors decide the questions put to them on the basis of their "intimate convic-tion" rather than by rigorous standards of proof, gave the panels many opportunities to render judgements that were not impartial.[1]

Likewise, in the Fiquet trial the process of deciding guilt or innocence, and of labeling and punishing the offender, was both intuitive and rational. Strong moral condemnation comes from a place of emotion, but so does mercy. Mitigation arises from an intuitive sense of natural justice, not just on the logical application of a code, which can result in injustice. To make this judg-ment call, the court needed to know what sort of woman Fiquet was. The statements contained in the dossier create a detailed portrait, but only some of this information was presented at the trial.

What was Marie-Françoise Fiquet like as a wife? Her marriage to Pierre Fiquet was an unhappy union. Her husband's fifteen-year-old niece, Marie Fenet, told the investigation in July 1882 that the femme Fiquet "mistreated her husband daily" and had admitted to the girl, "We have not had an inti-mate relationship together for over two years."[2] She made no secret of her affairs with other men. These included a sexual liaison with a mid-thirties Catholic priest, the Abbé Pihéry, in Besançon, where the Fiquet family had lived from 1879 to 1880 prior to their move to Dijon. The Catholic Church, although officially mandating the celibacy of priests, has only ever main-tained partial control over the sexual mores of its anointed. Historically, therefore, intimate relationships between priests and their parishioners have been common, and misbehaving priests were regularly satirized in European literature, from *The Canterbury Tales* to *The Decameron* and *The Héptameron*.[3]

The morality dossier contains ninety-four letters from the Abbé Pihéry, written to Marie-Françoise Fiquet between May 1879 and June 1880 (averaging two letters per week).[4] These date from the time she was living in Besançon, a town some ninety kilometers (fifty-six miles) west of Dijon, with her husband and daughter and their niece, the aforementioned Marie Fenet. On 15 July 1882, a fortnight after Henriette's murder, Pihéry gave a statement from his residence in the same town. Claiming he had only visited the family's home "once, maybe twice," Pihéry called the femme Fiquet a dishonest woman of "doubtful morality," though he declined to pass on the letters he had received from her, invoking the Seal of the Confessional.[5] Presumably this was convenient for Pihéry, because the investigators also had a note from the magistrate requesting information from two possible witnesses to the couple's alleged affair in Besançon: a police officer, named Magnin, and a bailiff, named Rabot. These two men were asked to confirm "in what circumstances they found (in the month of July 1879) the *femme* Fiquet lying down with a priest—what was their position in the bed, was the priest still wearing his robes, etc."[6]

In one of his letters to the femme Fiquet, dated 8 October 1879, Pihéry alluded to "intimate matters that it is better not to discuss in letters," and in his correspondence he regularly chastised Fiquet for being demanding: "As I told your niece, I cannot come up to your house today."[7] We might infer from this note that his visits were much more frequent than the one or two visits he claimed to have made. In the statements given in July 1882 by Marie Fenet, the teenager confirmed many important details about Fiquet's daily life and habits—most importantly, that she had been pregnant in 1879:

> I lived in Pierre Fiquet's house in Besançon for seven months in 1879. We lived in a little isolated house near the Chapelle des Buis. The *femme* Fiquet treated her husband very badly every day; he could not say a word without her getting angry. She constantly threatened him. . . . She didn't do any work, she was debauched, she received men at the house. I very frequently went to the pharmacists in town to get remedies for her, it was generally laudanum. Because she was indigent, she was given vouchers to obtain medicines for free. She would falsify the prescriptions the doctors provided to increase the dose. Sometimes she would go to get the medicines herself. As soon as she was back at home, she hurried to remove the label from the medicine bottle, she took these medicines through a straw that she placed in the bottle. All this happened at the time she was pregnant. Besides, she did not hide her pregnancy.[8]

In the same testimony, Fenet said that Fiquet received regular visits from a Jesuit priest (presumably Pihéry) who gave her money and who stayed a long time to hold "private conversations" with her. In her later testimony given in court in 1883, Fenet added that her aunt would undress and get into bed before the priest arrived and that he would go into Fiquet's bedroom.[9] One night in July 1879, recounted Fenet, "the *femme* Fiquet came to wake me around eleven o'clock in the evening, she handed me a sealed cotton bag. This bag was about the size of a bushel, she had me carry it to the river, and advised me to not speak of it, she had been sick for two or three days previously."

Marie Fenet testified that the femme Fiquet had been pregnant and then was no longer pregnant, so the "cotton bag" she described in all likelihood contained the remains of an infant—a late miscarriage, an abortion, or an early infanticide. The disposal of the bundle in a nearby waterway was a detail that foreshadowed the disposal of Henriette's body in the canal in Dijon, according to Fenet. Fiquet refused to speak of the events of that evening.[10] It is indeed plausible, then, that the Abbé Pihéry fathered a child that was later dispatched like a litter of newborn kittens. This incident would be invoked in the trial to suggest callousness on the part of Fiquet toward her unborn or recently born child: it would not be interpreted as an act of desperation or indeed as part of the everyday burden of exploitation carried by nineteenth-century working women.

Further documentation in the dossier suggests that this was not the first time Fiquet had lost an infant. Two notes, dated October 1882, confirmed that while still a teenager she had given birth to two illegitimate daughters, the second of whom had died. The first daughter, Marie-Louise, was born in 1869 and was thirteen in 1882 (this was the daughter, Louise, who had been legally adopted by Pierre Fiquet, though she was not his biological child) and would testify against her mother. The second girl, Marie-Emilie, was born in 1870 and died the following year.[11] The death of the femme Fiquet's second baby plausibly left a psychological wound to which she would return. We do not know how or why Marie-Emilie died nor why Marie-Louise lived.

If Fiquet remained silent on the liaison with the Abbé Pihéry, it is perhaps because she was never asked about it: Defendants had neither the right to know the exact nature of the accusation against them nor the right to see any evidence, and the priest's letters would later be classed as inadmissible evidence in court.[12] That her niece's testimony was not pursued beyond what it confirmed about Fiquet's past behavior is unsurprising, in a context in which female witnesses were often viewed as unreliable. Dominique Kalifa, for example, has argued that the purpose of the judicial inquiry in late nineteenth-century France was to "make the crime representable." A narrative had to be constructed with a logical shape to provide a compelling explanation. The role of women in these inquiries was strictly circumscribed: They appeared only as passive agents in a world that was inherently masculine and conservative.[13] Women also tended to be viewed in terms of their relationship to men—fathers, brothers, husbands—and therefore incapable of providing objective testimony.[14]

The suggestions of abortion or infanticide that would later be presented in Fiquet's trial would have been meaningful to a contemporary audience and fed directly into contemporary anxieties about depopulation that crystallized in the early decades of the twentieth century in France.[15] Abortion, which had been strictly repressed during the ancien régime under the influence of the Church, had been formally outlawed under article 317 of the 1810 penal code, which specified that any woman seeking an abortion and anyone helping her would be condemned to forced labor.[16] Although therapeutic abortion was a right recognized by the Academy of Medicine in 1852, the ethics of abortion became a topic of debate and controversy in the early 1900s. An editorial signed by seven prominent Parisian doctors and published in Le Matin on 26 December 1910 under the headline "Pour les Innocents" condemned the practice for the danger it posed to women and for the demoralization it produced in the wider population. The subtitle read, "The Academy of Medicine speaks out against the unwitting suicide of women and the ongoing murder of children."

Contemporary attitudes toward abortion varied, however (as they do today), and started to shift significantly from around 1890. Many notable writers and journalists, such as Victor Margueritte, a vocal defender of women's liberation, publicly stated their support for women's access to legal abortion.[17] These liberalizing attitudes fed into a backlash and anxieties about depopulation expressed by the doctors who wrote the piece in Le Matin. Historical demographer René Le Mée has argued that contemporary hospital records of deaths of young women for "gynecological" reasons, which went down in this period, suggest that rates of illicit abortion increased after 1870, while rates of infanticide fell. Le Mée attributes this shift to the evolution of medical techniques and abortion using medical instruments rather than noxious plant medicines. Although these new methods were far from safe, as revealed by the aforementioned death statistics, they were more effective, and many more midwives and doctors had become skilled in these new techniques.[18] It was in this context of increased medical professionalization that Marie-Françoise Fiquet came to be attracted to the career of midwifery.

The dossier also recorded the femme Fiquet's involvement in another sexual liaison, this time with a young medical intern, Dr. Michelot, who had treated Fiquet with morphine at her home in Dijon in 1880. According to a statement from the widow Barbey (the Fiquets' neighbor, and, coincidentally, Henriette's aunt), Fiquet was "in the habit of" receiving a young medical intern at her home and would "shut herself away for long periods of time" with him.[19] Since Marie Fenet had testified that her aunt had only ever taken laudanum solution in 1879, and the medical prescriptions found in the Fiquet home dated from 1880, it is likely that Fiquet's addiction to injected morphine began from this date. Marandon's medical report also recorded that the first administration of morphine was for severe back pain and had been given by a doctor named Professor Brulet in hospital in Dijon 1880.[20] The twenty-nine-year-old Dr. Michelot gave a statement to the police on 22 July 1882, in which he insisted that Fiquet was a deluded hysteric and that there had never been any relationship between them:

> It was in the month of July 1880 that I knew the *femme* Fiquet, from that time I saw her frequently in the hospital, where she would attend the consultation, she was even admitted to hospital several times, but she was not under my care. Her daughter who was about twelve years old was also admitted several times to hospital . . . so I often saw her mother. The *femme* Fiquet constantly said she was ill, she complained of violent headaches, she frequently used morphine, and in the hospital we quite often gave her subcutaneous injections of morphine, and each time she met me in the hospital or in the street, she insisted that I should go to administer the injections at her home, but I always refused.

After conceding that he did *once* go to her house (Fiquet had allegedly summoned him, pretending her daughter was ill), Michelot claimed that it was "a veritable pharmacy" containing syringes and bottles of morphine. In his statement, Michelot added that Fiquet had a reputation in the hospital as a "hypochondriac" who "kept all the services busy with her overbearing personality and her alleged illness. . . . This woman was a hysteric, she had fanciful ideas, she claimed to be unknown and misunderstood, that she was not in the right place. This woman was afflicted with some kind of mania, and I think I noticed that at times she did not seem to be in possession of her intellectual faculties."[21] Michelot's reference to Louise's undefined illnesses and admissions to hospital also look suspicious, with hindsight, in the context of a hypothesis of factitious disorder.

Michelot articulated something revealing here. Marie-Françoise Fiquet held the conviction that she deserved recognition and appreciation. She was ambitious and believed she could achieve these things. Ambition had long been pathologized as a presenting symptom among groups of people not culturally expected to exhibit this personality trait, such as women and members of the lower classes. Psychiatric concepts such as "ambitious monomania" and "delirium of grandeur" were labels applied to these ideas.[22] This brief comment demonstrated that questions of class and gender were at the center of Fiquet's disturbance. Her life was full of pain and drudgery, but she dreamed of being someone with status: was her addiction to transgressive behavior a means of laying claim to power and experiencing a thrill that took her beyond her everyday life?

Later medical reports would cast doubt on Michelot's assessment. Why was he the only doctor to believe Fiquet was mentally ill, when others considered her sane? Like the Abbé Pihéry, Michelot claimed he had only visited Fiquet's home on one occasion. Given the suggestion that Michelot had a brief affair with the femme Fiquet, he had every motive for discrediting her as a mad hysteric. Michelot's statement is, however, useful—even if it was not entirely truthful. He alluded to the same cluster of behaviors that would see Fiquet later diagnosed as a "simulator" of illness. His testimony intensified the view that she was a fantasist obsessed with medicine and human anatomy, and other witness statements would confirm this; while her husband and daughter were half-starved and dressed in rags, she spent all the housekeeping money on drugs and medical textbooks.[23]

As mentioned in Pierre Fiquet's statements, Marie-Françoise Fiquet's driving ambition had been to become a midwife. As the investigation discovered, she had enrolled in midwifery classes in Dijon, but fellow students and the teaching doctor described her as entirely unsuited to the course—she was an "alcoholic" and a "morphinomaniac" who was always falling asleep in lessons. She was described as *légère*—fickle, unserious, or of questionable morality.[24] On 3 July 1882, five days after Henriette's death, the *Côte-d'Or* reported that Fiquet had received training as a midwife but had not been admitted to the profession.[25]

The investigation also established that Fiquet had a reputation for ingratiating herself with vulnerable young pregnant women. The dossier contains records of a series of predatory attempts by Marie-Françoise Fiquet to act out her doomed fantasy of being or becoming a midwife. These desires were born, plausibly, from her own losses—as we have seen, that of Marie-Emilie, who died in 1871, and of a second baby in 1879, as noted in Marie Fenet's testimony.[26] Another of Fiquet's neighbors, Marie Cagnard, gave a detailed statement to police in which she described Pierre Fiquet as "harmless," an honest and decent man, but where she also noted that the femme Fiquet had once offered a woman named Parot an abortion.[27] Fiquet was also accused of molestation and giving inappropriate and harmful advice to an anxious, young pregnant woman, called Mademoiselle Bautut, who would later testify in the trial. Bautut described how the femme Fiquet had pretended to be a midwife, inappropriately touched her, and attempted an abortion without her consent.[28] Fiquet's alarming behavior led to her being ostracized even within the community of women in which she lived.

In 1898, Raymond de Ryckère devoted a chapter of his book *La Femme en prison* to condemning the scandal of infanticide and abortion, a phenomenon he blamed on pleasure-loving, "denatured women" who, using poverty or social shame as an "excuse," willingly handed over the fate of their babies to "shrews" who unscrupulously took money, ostensibly to care for them, and instead disposed of the infants. Ryckère declared this to be the female crime "par excellence," fitting woman's cowardly and cruel nature. He asserted that baby-killing occurred on an industrial scale in many contexts—citing cases from England, France, Italy, and elsewhere. Although they were cut from the same ideological cloth, Cesare Lombroso took a lighter view of abortion than Ryckère, viewing it as an incidental and widespread practice, while classifying infanticide as a crime of passion or an act of temporary insanity. For the Italian doctor these were not, in fact, signs of the "born criminal" but rather regrettable realities endemic to the life of the city.[29]

Criminal cases from the turn of the century showed that juries were often lenient in such cases because they sympathized with poor, socially marginalized women who killed their babies out of desperation.[30] Pregnancy, menstruation, and childbirth were seen as periods of great psychological instability. For example, Ruth Harris cites the case of a certain *femme* Charmillon who was accused of murdering her baby but acquitted on the grounds that the neonatal period caused her to go mad.[31]

Ryckère's view was a recapitulation of centuries-old suspicions held about the powers of women who worked as healers, midwives, and nurses. The traditional accusation of witchcraft leveled against women in these roles was a means of disciplining those who exercised power over matters of life and death. Women accused of witchcraft in earlier times were often lay healers who helped peasants deal with their daily pains and sufferings. Some scholars have further argued that there is continuity between the suppression of witches in medieval and early modern Europe and the rise of the medical profession in nineteenth-century America and Europe, which excluded women and prevented them from working as independent practitioners as they had for centuries. Because they disrupted women's capacity for reproduction, female healers and midwives were a threat to the male ruling classes, whether the Catholic Church or the bourgeois professions, and they were often politically dissident figures.[32]

Women who occupied these roles often represented a threat to power, and they exerted influence in their own ways—positively and, in the case of

Marie-Françoise Fiquet, negatively. Fiquet demonstrably exercised a form of power that exceeded the reach of the doctors, priests, and police who attempted to discipline her. She was a subversive force, who inflicted an invisible and difficult-to-detect harm: She was uncontrollable, lewd, sexually deviant, and an insult to the virtuous working classes. Her actions made it easy to cast the femme Fiquet as a dangerous outsider: She was a working-class woman on the margins of society, who "attended" to other women of her rank whose lives were invisible; she was ambitious and intellectually curious; she was ready to take life and had apparently freely chosen her actions, although later she would describe being driven by an irresistible "urge" that she could not clearly explain. Many women in this context operated with benign intentions; Fiquet's motivations were altogether more opaque.

For some social commentators, the behavior of unruly women like Marie-Françoise Fiquet was the reason the country was in crisis—women were not having enough babies and were not being good mothers.[33] Hannah Frydman's research on classified advertising in the back pages of the French press at the turn of the century, two decades after the Fiquet affair, has shown that the abortion business was quietly booming: "Women's commercial, nonmonogamous, and nonreproductive sexuality and commodified methods for its control could be found in even the most respectable, widely read newspapers, using coded but legible terms. . . . Such ads were so visible that Marie Roger, president of the Midwives' General Trade Union, felt the need to defend the profession against 'unflattering suppositions.' Under Roger's direction, the union pledged to eliminate these ads and restore honor to the name of the profession."[34] Despite the efforts of the Union, it would never be possible to disentangle the life-giving power of the midwife from her ability to also take life nor to illuminate the gray areas in between.

In 1881, Fiquet had met an unmarried girl, named only Franchinal in the report (fille Franchinal), at the maternity hospital in Dijon. It is not clear what reason Fiquet had for being there. This meeting would prove to be the reason Fiquet and her husband would later regularly visit their local cemetery. Franchinal had given birth to twin boys, who died soon after they were born. Fiquet claimed in her statements that her plan had been to adopt the twins.[35] As we have seen, according to her daughter, Louise, Fiquet had also pretended to her husband that she was the twins' mother. As Louise explained in a statement to the investigating magistrate:

> Last winter, I had gone with my father to my grandmother's house at Moissey. After we'd been there for a month, my mother wrote to tell us that she had given birth to twins and that we were to come home if we

wanted to see them. We came home, and we only found my mother lying in bed. She told my father that the children had been buried. But she told me that she had not given birth. My father still believes that he has two children in the cemetery and my mother sometimes takes him there to see the graves. If I am not mistaken . . . the graves are those of two children of a woman [the *fille* Franchinal] who gave birth at the maternity hospital.[36]

Louise Fiquet would later suggest that her adoptive father knew the twins were not his but that he believed Marie-Françoise had given birth to them.[37] This pretense led to a somber daily ritual for the couple, who would go to the cemetery in Dijon each afternoon to visit the grave of the Franchinal twins. As the cemetery warden, Claude Coupé, testified, "Last July I reported to the Commissaire de Police that some flowers had been stolen from one grave . . . and these flowers had been found placed on the grave of the Franchinal children, a grave that was secretly tended by the *femme* Fiquet."[38] This evidence adds to the wider picture of Fiquet as a woman psychologically marked by the loss of her own infants and who, as a result, developed a compulsion to interfere with other people's babies and children and to invest in surrogate grief, a fantasy into which she also drew her unsuspecting husband.

When the family apartment was searched following the death of Henriette Barbey, the police found eleven artificial porcelain flowers, four statuettes, and two medallions that had been stolen and hoarded to decorate the twins' grave.[39] In a later letter to Loiseau, the investigating magistrate, dated 22 October 1882, Fiquet explained that she liked to go to cemeteries because they were "sad and lonely places" where she could communicate with the dead, a reference to her interest in Spiritism, which will be investigated in further detail in chapter 4.[40]

Due to low birth weight and the increased instance of prematurity, perinatal deaths of twins were common even into the twentieth century, and there is no direct evidence that Fiquet caused the death of Franchinal's two baby boys. But her mournful attachment to the graves of children that were not hers seems unusual. Other documented female murderers did also use baby "adoption" as a stepping stone toward becoming mass infant killers. For example, notorious English murderess Amelia Dyer would be executed in 1896 for killing several infants she had accepted money to "adopt." In *La Femme en prison et devant la mort*, Ryckère noted that "adoption" was often a code word and euphemism, understood by both the abandoning mother and the "midwife" or "nurse" who was paid discreetly for the service, to indicate the intention to get rid of a child. Citing the shocking example of Victorian "baby farms," where "adopted" children were allegedly kept in a state of neglect and semistarvation until they died or were killed, Ryckère blamed the problem on unbridled female sexuality. Indeed, women who found themselves on the wrong side of the law often did so because they had harmed children.

Amelia Dyer is cited in Ryckère's tome as the prototypical "angel maker" that Fiquet was possibly in the process of becoming. Like Fiquet, the Englishwoman had spent long periods in hospital and was considered a self-dramatizing "simulator" of mental illness. Dyer also abused laudanum and habitually disposed of the bodies of infants in rivers and waterways near her home in Reading. Ryckère also maintained that religiosity, particularly when expressed by imprisoned women, was a key murderous trait, and applied to both Dyer and Fiquet. In Fiquet's case, her belief in spirit guides dominated the account she gave of her own actions.

A strikingly similar case to that of Amelia Dyer in France has been highlighted by Odile Krakovitch in her research into the transportation of women to the French penal colonies. In 1867, a woman named Victoire Veysseyre, a midwife, "baby farmer," and wet nurse, was found guilty of having "disappeared" up to six children in her care. In a particularly grisly example, she was found to have locked two newborn babies in a suitcase during an entire coach journey from Le Puy to Saint-Étienne, during which time they died. Veysseyre was also suspected of having poisoned her husband's first wife and of killing his daughter through abuse and neglect. The accused woman was condemned to death, though the sentence was commuted to hard labor; she was transported to Nouméa, New Caledonia, where she lived to the age of seventy-eight. The case was reported at length in the *Gazette des Tribunaux*, which described in painful detail the gratuitous cruelty, horrific neglect, and suffering inflicted on a two-year-old child found in her "care" who immediately died from her injuries and infections. The femme Veysseyre was described as a sociopath who demonstrated "hatred for human existence," such was the depravity of her behavior.[41]

Ruth Homrighaus's research on the care of illegitimate children in England found that a quarter of the thirty-two female murderers executed for their crimes after 1870 were baby farmers.[42] The reality of baby farming, however, as Homrighaus has shown, was more varied and shaded with gray than the stereotypes promoted by commentators like Ryckère: "At a time when neither the government nor private philanthropists provided adequately for the children of impoverished unmarried women, baby farming evolved as an uncoordinated but functional range of strategies for coping with and capitalizing on the existence of unwanted infants."[43] Baby farming was a structural solution to the complex problem of infant care for women who needed to work. It ranged from paying women to legitimately nurse children to giving up babies for "adoption" to unscrupulous people, whose motives were unclear. Some infants were well cared for; others were neglected or abused or even killed. Notorious cases that came to light through criminal proceedings meant that so-called baby farmers earned a negative reputation and became the focus of campaigns to outlaw the practice.[44]

Margaret Waters, an English baby farmer convicted and hanged in October 1870 for causing the deaths of infants in her care, was cast in contemporary press reports as a monster who deserved her fate. The reality was more complex, and there is evidence that she did feed the babies and administer conventional treatments (according to the norms of the era). But abandoned infants who were not wet-nursed simply did not have a good chance of survival. It is noteworthy, given the details of the Fiquet case, that Waters was also accused of administering laudanum to babies to sedate them when hungry or unsettled for other reasons. It is far from clear, however, that Waters deliberately killed the infants. The practice of baby farming troubled public opinion because it showed that infanticide was not just an act committed by a desperate mother but rather a business that held up a mirror to a society in which the bonds of kinship had been fractured. It was the very definition of vice, as the reversal of traditional virtue. Women willing to deal with unwanted babies, even to the point of causing their deaths, believed they were doing good. Many of them agreed that if a child was born to a single woman in poverty, it was better off not surviving. The fact that some women were willing to deal with this reality challenged conventional ideas about feminine nurture and nonviolence.[45]

Homrighaus's thesis is compelling, but it also assumes rational motives on the part of women who set themselves up as baby farmers. They were responding to a genuine need and providing a service for which there was significant demand. However, the Fiquet case, among others, illustrates that individual psychology also entered the picture. Plausibly, psychologically disturbed or personality disordered women with issues around control, illness, and death would be drawn to operate in unsupervised contexts that allowed them to care for vulnerable infants. Not all were bad actors, but some clearly were, and many would have been a bit of both. The femme Fiquet, for example, clearly held the capacity to nurture, but her destructive behavior seemed to have been an extension or twisting of her desire to care—for example, in the possible administration of morphine to Henriette Barbey.

Marie-Françoise Fiquet also fantasized about "treating" people with drugs, and the dossier contains circumstantial evidence that she had killed before.

There are two statements relating to suspicious incidents, the first concerning a girl named Vacherot who had been given "remedies" by the femme Fiquet and subsequently died, apparently of meningitis.[46] Another witness, the femme Vauthier, who resided at 12 rue Musette, gave a statement in which she claimed to have had "an instinctive aversion towards" her neighbor, the femme Fiquet, who had taken care of an old spinster and Spiritist, Mademoiselle Vallangin, until her death. According to Vauthier, the old woman had been terrified of Fiquet. These accusations would be cited again in the press reporting of the trial, with the lawyer for the prosecution claiming, "Two years ago, in your home you treated a certain Miss Valangin [sic], who was a Spiritist. This woman died and you stole everything from her, even her clothes. There were serious rumors—there was talk of poisoning."[47] Gossip that had circulated at the time was leveraged by the prosecution as strong circumstantial evidence of Fiquet's poor character.

The accusations of poisoning would continue. As mentioned in the Fiquets' own statements, three weeks prior to Henriette Barbey's abduction, Pierre Fiquet had been suffering from an unexplained sickness. His neighbors' concern at his condition had been such that between them they had paid for a carriage to take him to hospital; he only returned home to the rue Musette on the day of Henriette's abduction.[48] On 4 July, Louise Fiquet told the investigation that her mother had resisted him being taken to hospital. Two days later, Dr. Deroye confirmed that he had been called to treat Pierre Fiquet, who was suffering with vomiting, diarrhea, and burning in the throat.[49] These symptoms—and the femme Fiquet's suspicious behavior—led several neighbors to accuse her of having attempted to poison her husband. In Louise's account, her mother all but admitted her culpability: "My mother had no affection for my father. When he was ill, she would give him bouillon that she went to buy. I don't know if she put anything in it. She said that on no account should my father be taken to hospital . . . that he had no more than eight days to live. . . . She also told me that if my father were to die in hospital, that she would be thrown to the dogs."[50]

These accounts suggest that the killing of Henriette Barbey formed part of a larger pattern of quietly violent behavior for Marie-Françoise Fiquet, who had almost certainly been poisoning her husband. These stereotypically female forms of "gentle" aggression appear to have included infanticide and abortions, poisoning and the administering of potentially fatal medicines, and eventually drowning. These actions, considered alongside Fiquet's fascination with medical professions and her psychiatrists' suggestions that she simulated illness, point to the conclusion that hers was an early case of what would later be called Munchausen syndrome (and Munchausen syndrome

by proxy), now more commonly categorized under the umbrella of factitious personality disorder.

Of course, not all women who lose infants develop the destructive behaviors that Fiquet exhibited. Unique to this case, and to some analogous cases
already mentioned, was the translation of this initial trauma into violence—
producing the libidinal satisfaction gained from the harmful but not deadly
desire to induce or fabricate illness—and the slippage between this and the
act of killing. It has been observed that people with the psychological capacity to kill repeatedly in this way are often attracted to working within medical settings that give them the opportunity to act on their impulses. These
so-called angels of death can be male or female, although the image is often
coded female due to the incongruence between caring and nurturing and
violence.[51] Central to these cases is the element of repetition and the aura of
suspicion that hangs around perpetrators until they are caught, which was
clearly manifested in Fiquet's case.

In an analysis of a parallel set of cases that occurred a generation later, of
a group of Hungarian women who poisoned dozens of men in the region
of Tiszazug between 1911 and 1929, Béla Bodó has argued that quietly violent behaviors such as poisoning and infanticide were intimately connected
and were generally carried out by women because of the heavily gendered
structures of peasant society.[52] Bodó has demonstrated that these extreme
methods offered a means for women to resolve untenable social pressures.
Sick, elderly relatives in need of nursing care and hungry infants were generally a problem for mothers and daughters, not fathers and sons.

Women in peasant society also traditionally held the important functions
of nurses, healers, cooks, and carers. The rigid entrenchment of gender
roles in early twentieth-century Hungarian peasant communities meant that
women and men lived separately from childhood and maintained separate
cultures. Women faced unique problems, resorted to other women for help,
and as caregivers could easily assume the role of aggressor under extreme
pressure. The brutality of conditions in this society meant that child neglect
and infanticide were relatively common, and people were unsentimental
about the weak. Significantly, the leading woman in the case had been the
village midwife, who had been imprisoned for performing illegal abortions.

Bodó does, however, insist that the Tiszazug murders were exceptional:
They did *not* form part of a wider, accepted peasant culture for dealing with
the weak, in the same way that Fiquet's reaction to her losses was in some
sense outside the norm. A contextualizing explanation does not amount to
a generalization. This view was reflected in the contemporary reporting of
the Tiszazug killings in the British press, which viewed them as aberrant and

motivated by financial greed.[53] Both the Hungarian peasant murders and the Fiquet affair were interpreted in contemporary sources as being out of the ordinary, but there are commonalities to the stresses they foregrounded.

I would suggest the pattern was similar. Marie-Françoise Fiquet and the Hungarian peasant midwives were cynical and self-interested women who were prepared to take serious risks. They attempted something exceptional that to most people would be beyond the pale and even terrifying. Having escaped without detection or punishment once or twice, they became hooked on the thrill of playing a game of life and death—one that was also to their financial advantage.

In light of the infamous Marie Lafarge affair, the poison law in France had been changed in 1845 to restrict access to potentially deadly substances.[54] Reactions to this earlier case showed that husband poisoners were held to be particularly aberrant and were greatly feared, because almost every man in France could be a potential target.[55] The controversy over this case centered on the perceived disconnect between Lafarge's outwardly respectable character and the apparent murder of her husband, by giving him food laced with arsenic, for which she was later found guilty. Marie Lafarge was subsequently cited by Lombroso in 1893 as an example of the female inborn criminal. As Lisa Downing has argued, "The concern with Marie's guilt or innocence served to cover a different concern of modern society: an anxiety about gender roles and especially the incompatibility of narrow cultural perceptions of feminine nature with acts that are assertive, aggressive, or violent and, simultaneously, the equally persistent, troubling fantasy that women may in fact embody exactly these qualities."[56]

Though abortion was, to an extent, tacitly tolerated in nineteenth-century France, homicide by poisoning (or the attempt to do so) was considered a particularly heinous, cruel, and cowardly crime. It was accorded a special category in the penal code because it was so difficult to detect. After parricide, deemed the most unnatural act of violence and a capital crime, and poisoning, murdering a child was considered a most aberrant crime against the womanly, nurturing instinct. The accusation of poisoning on the part of the femme Fiquet would have therefore been a revelation loaded with meaning for a courtroom audience, and the unproven allegations of poisoning, abduction, and abortion (or infanticide) would have carried great cultural significance: No woman was executed in France between 1905 and 1943. The last woman to be guillotined, during the Second World War under the Vichy regime, was condemned to death for carrying out abortions.[57] Although abortion was not a capital offense under the early Third Republic in 1883, it was clearly a significant, recurring cultural issue, and the law would shift to emphasize the differences in public opinion that existed.

The rumors that circled around the femme Fiquet, together with evidence of her preoccupation with contacting the dead, led the investigation to pursue the hypothesis that Marie-Françoise Fiquet was the principal author of the crime. She had acted without a comprehensible motive, and her husband was perceived to be a passive and powerless accomplice who deserved a lesser punishment. The dominant view outside the investigation was more lenient still, considering Pierre Fiquet to be an imbecilic victim who had himself narrowly avoided being murdered by his wife. This leniency would later be shown in court, when Mr. Fiquet's defense lawyer, Paul Cunisset, asserted that his client was "under the influence of this woman who viewed him merely as a slave."[58]

As we have seen, Fiquet was darkly fascinated with anatomy and medicine, and she played out a long and fatal game of control over the arbitrary forces of nature, sickness, life, and death. Several triggers led to the abduction and death of Henriette Barbey as the culmination of these disturbed fantasies. First, the femme Fiquet's ambition to practice midwifery was again thwarted: On 24 June 1882, just a few days before she abducted Henriette, she had received a letter from the mayor of Moissey, a small town halfway between Dijon and Besançon, politely declining her offer to work there as a midwife.[59] Second, her husband, whom she had failed to poison, returned home from hospital. Finally, as previously mentioned, and as the evidence from the statement given by the silversmith Schettine confirmed, Fiquet's syringe was broken and she was therefore in morphine withdrawal. These stresses led Marie-Françoise Fiquet to abruptly leave her job at the tobacco factory, without ever giving a reason.[60] The following day, 29 June 1882, would be the day to again act out her destructive fantasies, but this time she would leave an indelible trace of her actions from which she could no longer flee.

CHAPTER 4

The Medical Reports

When interrogated, Marie-Françoise Fiquet paradoxically claimed to have acted under *both* the influence of drugs *and* the stress of morphine withdrawal. She also claimed to be guided by spirits and to have acted on a mysterious and uncontrollable impulse. In cases where delirium was suspected, it was standard protocol to bring in medicolegal experts to assess the extent of the subject's criminal responsibility.[1] In 1882, even in a provincial town like Dijon, a crime as rare and serious as child murder warranted a psychiatric investigation.

Seven weeks after her arrest, Fiquet was duly placed in the Chartreuse asylum in Dijon, in the service of Dr. Évariste Marandon de Montyel, where she would be observed from 17 August to 15 October 1882. The rationale for this decision was based on Fiquet's self-reporting of nervous illness:

In the presence of a woman who said she had been affected by serious nervous and other illnesses, who had frequently stayed in hospitals, who had consulted many doctors and who claimed to have had mental blanks caused by the abuse of opiate medicines, the investigating magistrate thought it was his duty to submit the accused woman to a continued and prolonged medical observation, and, upon his orders, the *femme* Fiquet was placed in the Chartreuse asylum, around the middle of August, and she stayed there until 15 October.[2]

Marandon, in his early thirties, was a medical director who reported being intimidated by the responsibility of assessing the femme Fiquet, even though the case seemed clear-cut, as he later recalled, "I still found the task I was called upon to complete too weighty for my young shoulders to bear."[3] Marandon was perhaps an unorthodox choice. Such cases were usually taken by experienced and distinguished Parisian psychiatrists, and Marandon was not yet a medico-legal specialist, and he was certainly not famous.[4] However, as an up-and-coming medical director, he was considered sufficiently qualified. The young physician accepted the challenge and would go on to have a distinguished career as director of the psychiatric service at the Ville-Évrard asylum in Neuilly-sur-Marne and later as director of public asylums in the Seine region.[5]

Marandon would be best remembered for his (largely unsuccessful) attempts to introduce an "open door" method into French asylums. This aimed to end the "dangerous and painful" practice of isolating mental patients within asylum-prisons. In Marandon's vision, asylums would be more like farms, in which residents would have the opportunity to work outside on the land and would be free to move around under the supervision of asylum superintendents.[6] As Jessie Hewitt has indicated, Marandon and other advocates of this method were progressive alienists with a less hierarchical vision of the doctor-patient relationship than both their predecessors and many of their contemporaries, who emphasized moral treatment and the containment of incurable degenerates.[7]

Some legal experts have pointed out that psychiatry, when used in the courtroom, tends to be shrouded in mystery and characterized by a certain "untouchability."[8] Mental illness can be diagnosed only through the identification of symptoms, and the framing of behavior as disease requires an interpretive act that defines it as such—madness, or irresponsibility, versus badness or willing wickedness. Since the femme Fiquet had used her morphine habit to "excuse" her crime, and claimed to be possessed by spirits driving her to the scaffold, the role of the examining doctors was primarily to establish whether "morphinomania," or addiction to medical morphine, was the key to solving the mystery of what had been an otherwise motiveless murder or if it could be argued that she was clinically insane and under the influence of "voices," as she claimed.[9]

Marandon's professional opinion would be that Fiquet was a "simulator": She was neither mentally ill (aliénée) nor extremely affected by her morphine habit. However, he did infer from his observations of her behavior that Fiquet's pathological personality, of which her "passion" for morphine was symptomatic, and "her weak character, volatile thinking and lack of judgment" constituted grounds for the attenuation of criminal responsibility.[10]

The study of morphine addiction, or *morphinomanie*, was still at an embryonic stage in 1882, which makes the Fiquet case particularly interesting and important. Most major medical treatises on the subject—and therefore emerging conceptions of addiction—were published in the mid to late 1880s and 1890s.[11] In the early 1880s, Marandon therefore struggled to explain the crime within the framework of drug addiction. This hesitancy in his medical report on the Fiquet case produced a circularity in the narrative, which opened and closed with assertions regarding the confounding mystery surrounding his patient and equivocated on the question whether the femme Fiquet was mentally disturbed or simply morally evil.[12]

Marandon's report dealt with this uncertainty by overstabilizing elements of the story using a superficially neat medical gloss of an essentially incoherent and inexplicable event. It did not, however, make sense of the meaning and power of drug addiction and the psychological complexity of Fiquet's inner life. Her primary symptom of "simulation" was viewed as a counterindication of illness. The purpose of the medical reports was to prove that there was nothing that made Fiquet do what she did—not morphine, not delusions, not spirit possession—and therefore to show that, despite her heightened suggestibility and bizarre behavior, she could be held responsible for her crime.

These argumentative contortions were present in other contemporaneous cases of criminal women. In 1890, Gabrielle Bompard would be accused of being an accomplice to Michel Eyraud in the gruesome murder of Montmartre resident and bailiff Toussaint-Augustin Gouffé. Bompard was examined by a medicolegal team headed by the doyen of French forensic medicine, Paul Brouardel, who tested Bompard's past as a hypnotism subject. Although they found that she could be made to do anything under posthypnotic suggestion, they also managed to make their report fit with Jean-Martin Charcot's dictum that no one could commit a crime while thus hypnotized.[13]

The Bompard case was reported in the British periodical *The Spectator*, which criticized the behavior of the judge and the procureur-général, who conducted the case and who, "by dint of bullying the prisoners and by dwelling upon every sensational detail of the evidence, has contrived to give the proceedings a specially revolting character."[14] Although Bompard was not acquitted, her high level of suggestibility was considered mitigation, and she was spared the guillotine (Eyraud was executed for the murder) and sentenced to twenty years of hard labor. The courts did therefore consider female suggestibility and moral lability grounds for sufficient reasonable doubt to trigger a lesser sentence.

The 1880s were a crucial period in the evolution of medicolegal under-standings of crime as viewed through a scientific lens. The medical reports written on Fiquet's crime and her state of mind formed part of an emerging field of study. In anthropological criminology, dominated by Cesare Lom-broso and Alexandre Lacassagne by the later decades of the nineteenth cen-tury, there was a focus on the significance of physiognomy and the criminal body. But there was also growing interest in the ways in which criminals accounted for their actions, motives, and desires through their speech and writing. Psychiatric work on writing by patients also inspired criminologists to peer into the mind of the offender in a similar way.[15] In 1893, the role of medical experts in legal proceedings was formalized via a decree providing lists of medico-legists residing in the vicinity of each city court.[16] This branch of medical expertise was therefore not yet in its heyday when Fiquet was tried.

As Foucault showed in the Pierre Rivière dossier, the role of expert wit-nesses was to create a logical picture of a murderer. However, this picture did not always make clear sense and sometimes risked producing tensions between expert discourses. The internal contradictions in the medical argu-ments, which will be analyzed here, compounded the inconclusive nature of the case.

Marandon minimized or did not believe Fiquet's accounts of her physical pain, psychological disturbance, and struggles with morphine addiction. He saw Fiquet's "simulations" as evidence of her soundness of mind rather than symptoms of a generalized syndrome. The labeling of Fiquet as a simula-tor aligned with contemporary beliefs concerning the behavior of male and female murderers once apprehended. Ryckère, for example, put it plainly: "Men confess; women deny."[17] Gide's depictions of men facing justice were also striking for their insistence on the simplicity of the confession and the guilty owning their crimes.[18]

Irrespective of their aims or purpose, the medical reports foregrounded the voice of the femme Fiquet and retrospectively provide the reader with detailed and compelling information about the life she had led and the account she gave of her actions. They also offer a striking example of the medicolegal logic of the era. Written later than the original investigative records held in the dossier de procédure, and based in part on its contents, the medical reports offer a retelling of the case, beginning with the glossing of the witness statements from the dossier. Added to this were direct observa-tions of the accused woman's speech, writing, and behavior in detention at the asylum and in prison.

The Marandon Report

Marandon's report was first written for the investigating magistrate and was later published in the leading medical journal *L'Encéphale* in 1883. The title focused on the question of "morphinomania," but the main body of the report also foregrounded Fiquet's deceitful character and her use of both simulation and dissimulation to deflect responsibility for the death of Henriette. Marandon began, "I will seek to find out if morphinomania explains the mystery in which this double crime has remained shrouded." The alienist's mission, as he stated it, was "to find out if the drug altered her state of mind to such an extent that she lost the ability to act with good judgement."[19] Marandon argued that the effect of intoxicants varied from one person to another and that conclusions on someone's mental state could only be drawn by observing their "actions and words." He argued that *morphinomanie* was not a form of madness but an affliction born of habit and "reasoned imitation," by which he meant social contagion or the power of suggestion.[20]

Marandon believed that, because the femme Fiquet was a proven fraud and liar, there was "no possible doubt about the mental state of the accused."[21] Fiquet was troubled, but she was sane, because an insane person could not, it was assumed, make rational decisions. This claim set the tone for the whole medical investigation, which did not note any link between Fiquet's suffering and her addictive and destructive behavior. Marandon hinted at this idea when citing his predecessor, Bénédict Augustin Morel, known for his work on degeneration theory, who had argued that "all [addicts] seek in an artificial exaltation, full of charms, happiness if possible, and at least the forgetting of their sorrows."[22] Marandon's reference to Morel suggests he was aware of something beyond medical addiction that kept Fiquet dependent on morphine; however, he was conflicted on the question of how much this affected her free will.

The report began with the known details of Fiquet's poor character, and in this sense repeated the aims of the criminal investigation rather than offering a dispassionate assessment of the "morphinomania" under examination. Fiquet had, like some other poor working-class women, according to Marandon, "prostituted herself" at the age of fifteen, leaving "a deplorable reputation" wherever she went.[23] The young woman was described as a girl of "loose morals," as intelligent, manipulative, and attention seeking. Marandon instinctively judged the femme Fiquet as a woman who had deviated from the ideals of the virtuous working classes; this attitude was repeated in the press reporting of the case. In reality, the dividing line between poor, working women and prostitutes was so blurred as to almost not be a line at all, since so many engaged in occasional or clandestine prostitution when necessary, for survival.[24] Marandon's focus on morality, however, reflected common ideas about ideal womanhood and also showed a concern to disentangle what could be attributed to preexisting temperament and what could be shown to be the effects of morphine abuse.

Marie-Françoise Fiquet's peculiarity lay in her studied simulation of a range of illnesses, which often convinced doctors, who, as Marandon explained, "needed a great deal of patience and discernment in order to bring to light her duplicity." This was not a case of hypochondria or malingering but rather of feigned illness motivated by attention seeking, "an area that she fully exploited out of laziness and self-interest."[25] Fiquet's "self-interest" included a fierce professional ambition to access the medical world as a midwife. Marandon noted that her problematic behaviors—cheating, lying, and medical attention seeking—were well established before her morphine addiction became an issue and that they continued afterward: "The morphinomania of the *femme* Fiquet did not take away her deceitful behavior or her ability to manipulate others, neither did it temper her morals."[26]

For the prosecution to demonstrate that Fiquet was criminally responsible, it was necessary to falsify her claim of being absolutely under the influence of drugs. Therefore, Fiquet's claim to have acted out of character under morphine amnesia was logically presented as part of a wider picture of simulation of illness that predated the crime. The medical report noted that she initially insisted it was morphine's stupefying effect rather than the effect of withdrawal that had caused her to act strangely that day.[27]

Although Fiquet's claim to have been in a morphine haze was treated with skepticism, Marandon did not find a better explanation for her behavior. The motive for abducting and killing the child remained a puzzle. Fiquet's claim also contradicted earlier evidence about being in morphine withdrawal, although she did take a mixture of different drugs (including chloroform and the morphine solution) during the days when she was without her syringe, so it seems plausible that she was, indeed, *both* under the influence *and* in partial withdrawal from her usual morphine dose. At least, her usual means of administration had been disrupted.

The conclusion reached by the experts and in due course the jury, that neither addiction nor withdrawal explained Fiquet's actions, was in line with contemporary thinking on drug addiction and crime. Although withdrawal was a mitigating factor in many criminal cases, it was not enough to excuse murder, and intoxication itself was not generally viewed as an attenuating circumstance, due, as noted, to the observably pacifying and regulating effects of opiates.[28]

Fiquet's libido was paralleled in the report with her appetite for drugs, which she had shown a talent for acquiring without cost to herself via the city's charitable services. Marandon said that Fiquet also sold drugs, claiming it had been "proven" that she had illegally resold medicines that she had acquired for free. Fiquet, he explained, had developed a "passion for morphine" after being given the drug as a pain killer. All the doctors who examined her (eleven medical men would appear in court to testify against her),[29] agreed that Fiquet was deceitful, unscrupulous, and lazy yet also intelligent and fully aware of her actions even before she entered a period of "morphinic intoxication."[30] Despite the medical profession's ultimate responsibility for intoxicating Fiquet, the problematic morphine use—denoted via the morally loaded French terms *passion* and *ivrognerie* ("drunkenness")—was attributed to her defective character rather than medical addiction. Marandon maintained that Fiquet was in possession of her critical faculties.

Marandon treated Fiquet's claim to take a gram of morphine per day with skepticism, but this was entirely plausible. Marandon devoted a full page of the report to other historical accounts of unusually high doses of opiates, but he still disbelieved Fiquet.[31] There are two possible reasons for this. First, he examined his charge after she had withdrawn from morphine and her physical state was generally poor, making it difficult for him to tell whether her condition was due to morphine abuse or other factors:

> In the asylum, I focused my attention as much on her physical as her mental state; on the physical side, the accused woman was aged thirty-one, brown-haired, small, with a normal-shaped head, a blotchy face, and both arms covered in needle marks, lively and intelligent eyes, she presented above all with gastro-intestinal problems that were linked to her morphine habit. She ate very little, had difficulty digesting and often vomited her food and had almost continual diarrhea. She constantly complained of feeling thirsty and having headaches. Right up until the beginning of October she was covered in foul-smelling sweat, despite almost daily baths.[32]

His patient also suffered with insomnia, and despite arguing that she exaggerated them, Marandon conceded that these physical problems "could also have been real" and painted a wretched physical portrait of the woman.[33] Second, Marandon argued at some length that morphine was not a stronger intoxicant than alcohol or tobacco, nor more significant than a penchant for gambling or womanizing, and its effects insufficient to change someone's fundamental character.

To illustrate this claim he cited German physician Eduard Levinstein's examples of high-functioning addicts in the scientific and medical professions to argue that it was possible to maintain a morphine habit, act normally, and make ethical judgments: "I know a whole series of people who are morphinomaniacs to a high degree, and who find themselves in full possession of their intellectual vigor, who were or still are the most brilliant stars on the scientific horizon."[34] But Marandon did distinguish, with reference to other treatises on morphine abuse, between morphine addicts experiencing euphoria (*en puissance*) and withdrawal (*en abstinence*). He also acknowledged the well-documented distinction between those who had only recently started using the drug and the physically dependent who had developed long-term habits.[35]

Marandon argued that "euphoric" drug users were criminally responsible, whereas those at an extreme level of dependency might experience *le delirium tremems*, which Brouardel compared to opium visions, and therefore be "incapable of any reflection, of any planning."[36] Essentially, Marandon was arguing that someone in acute withdrawal could be in a state of mental agitation and even delusion and would therefore be incapable of premeditation and unable to execute a plan. The evidence of premeditation in the Fiquet case, for the observing doctor, precluded this possibility: "Applying these findings to the *femme* Fiquet, we see that the kidnapping and killing of Henriette Barbey, premeditated and cleverly executed, have absolutely no relation to morphinomania."[37]

Marandon argued that some attenuation of responsibility was reasonable in cases of addicts in withdrawal, but only if their actions were "demented or maniacal."[38] Yet, although it was clearly stated in the report that Fiquet *was* in withdrawal because her syringe was being repaired when the murder took place, Fiquet's actions on that day were not judged to be those of a maniac.[39] In order to square this argumentative circle, it was necessary to minimize the extent of the femme Fiquet's morphine use—and therefore of her potential withdrawal symptoms—by treating her claims of dependency with great skepticism.

As we have seen, Marandon at this time considered morphine use to be similar to alcohol and tobacco use and claimed that "morphinomania is a passion . . . which considered alone, has no medico-legal significance."[40] He had observed other cases of morphine dependency and concluded that it did not lead to dysregulation or murderous behavior. This study of *morphinomanie* was an emerging field, and clinical professionals, like Marandon, in 1882 lacked a secure conceptual framework within which to scrutinize the case. In the 1880s and 1890s, a high proportion of morphine addicts were male doctors, so Marandon would likely have seen high-functioning addicts working within his own profession.[41]

Although Marandon asserted that morphine habits could be controlled, he paradoxically used the image of the notoriously untamable femme fatale to evoke the allure of the drug, which he described as a seductive siren with a devil's tail: "After reasoned imitation comes the most dangerous means of spreading [morphinomania]: hearing morphine addicts praising the ineffable voluptuousness of their beloved drug, attracted by curiosity, enticed especially by the prospect of unknown pleasures, others followed them, reckless travelers who let themselves be enticed by the voice and deceitful charms of the siren, their eyes unable to see through the treacherous waters to see the forked tail of the monster beneath the waves."[42] The potency of the siren metaphor undermined Marandon's assertions about the irrelevance of morphine use to the question of criminal responsibility. The doctor resolved this tension by asserting that, although some people were powerless to control their addictions, the femme Fiquet was in control. Deprived of her "poison," he observed, she went into withdrawal at the clinic and experienced only mild symptoms. For Marandon, "this proves definitively that the accused woman was not as much of a morphinomaniac as she said."[43]

Marandon's attitude to his object of study was one of ambivalence and mild confusion. Fiquet possessed negative and positive traits, being sexually alluring, crafty, and intelligent but also menacing and quietly dangerous. Accordingly, she combined vice (deceit and laziness) with impressive personal qualities (intelligence and reason): "For all six doctors, the *femme* Fiquet was therefore a clever and deceitful woman, without scruples and magnificently lazy, but also very intelligent, in full possession of her mental faculties."[44] These contradictions would later be highlighted in the trial reports, which maintained that Fiquet was morally defective yet also intelligent, proving herself to be the intellectual match of the judge and other men in the courtroom. As Anna Norris has shown, these ambivalent attitudes were not uncommon in the period and reflected the assertions of Lombroso and Ryckère, as previously mentioned, who accounted for extreme female violence by claiming that women were morally inferior to men but capable of deploying their intelligence in the service of evil acts.[45] Women were doubly exceptional because they broke biological and social norms. These observations were similar to later descriptions of personality disorders in women.

A significant element of Fiquet's pathology was, according to Marandon, simply her brazenness. She acted entirely without compunction, which made it difficult for those examining her to feel sympathy for the woman.

For example, Marandon cast Fiquet's exploitation of Catholic and Protestant charitable resources as a mark of "irreverence" for the two religions, and her shamelessness made her "capable of anything."[46]

According to Marandon, only three out of the eleven doctors who had previously treated Fiquet observed any disturbance in her mental state. "One noticed something abnormal in the character of the accused woman, another that she had a strange manner. But [these] do not constitute madness." Only Michelot, the medical intern who treated Fiquet at home, discerned signs of a deeper possible mental disturbance: According to him, Fiquet "claimed to be misunderstood, ignored, and that she did not occupy the position in the world that she deserved."[47] Michelot's observation revealed that Fiquet's attitude was rooted in loss, a reaction to the indifference of the world to her ambitions. It supports the hypothesis that she exhibited a factitious disorder, which is usually driven by a need for recognition and attention from others. Indeed, Fiquet's apparent intelligence and her failed attempts to enter the profession of midwifery were signs of a deep desire to attract both medical attention and status in a class-ridden society in which her intellectual potential could not be realized in a conventional way.

Marandon also identified these same attention-seeking and perverse behaviors in a discussion of Fiquet's relationship with her husband:

> She was at pains to claim that, under the influence of morphine, she had lost her memory and found herself in a hazy mental state through which bizarre ideas came to her, like the idea of taking a little girl she had never seen before and who was passing by in the street, or that of falsely announcing to her absent husband the birth of two twins, even though they had not slept together in three years. . . . Judging by the behavior of Mr. Fiquet, he believed he was the father; indeed, he went to the cemetery and in the period that followed and continued to visit a little tomb that his wife had shown him. Marie Rémond [Fiquet] deeply detested her husband; she made him do all the most arduous chores, she not only made him hand over everything he earned, but also encouraged him to steal and repaid his guilty compliance with insults and insufficient food. A doctor, sent by the railway company to see the poor man suffering from appalling stomach pains, which got worse each time he took the bouillon prepared by his wife, was convinced that he was being poisoned, and despite Fiquet's energetic protests, had the sick man transported to hospital where he recovered without treatment in a few days. That woman was willing to do anything to torture the man who had married her despite her debauchery

and who had legally recognized a child born five years before their first relations. I see in this story a cruel wickedness and not an indication of madness.[48]

Marandon ruled out psychological disturbance and concluded that Fiquet's behavior was based in wicked opportunism. It is noteworthy that she refers here to her own "bizarre ideas" and her experience of an irresistible urge to abduct children. This reference to an intangible drive suggests there was a libidinal element to her behavior. The classic psychoanalytic view of perversion is that unresolved trauma is revisited psychically by the person affected and that it can be sexualized. This results in two things: first, a compulsion to repeat, and second, the temporary achievement of pleasure and satisfaction from the act. In Fiquet's case, she seemed to be conveying the idea that her life was banal and insignificant. She craved excitement and recognition, and abducting or acquiring children that were not hers, in replacement of those she had lost, was perhaps an addictive solution to her frustration.

The conclusion of the first part of Marandon's investigation was therefore that Fiquet was not truly mentally disturbed prior to gaining her morphine habit. None of the witnesses in the case noticed what might have been construed as "moral insanity" in the femme Fiquet, only that she was a wicked and self-interested woman. Marandon found Fiquet's claimed amnesia and experience of dissociation to be fraudulent, and he concluded that because her actions were premeditated, they could not have been caused by the influence of drugs: "These are the facts, and they clearly establish that the act was willed, planned and skillfully executed."[49]

Marandon's report also reproduced two of Fiquet's letters in which she discussed her Spiritist beliefs and her claim to be possessed, and which hint again at the power of the repetition compulsion and irresistible urge she experienced. The first letter had been sent by Fiquet to the examining magistrate from the Chartreuse asylum on 10 November 1882, and it was urgently forwarded to Marandon back at the asylum as possible evidence of mental disturbance. In the text, the "spirit" and morphine seem to be interchangeable ideas that Fiquet used to explain her violent actions on the day she had abducted her final victim.

I have something to say to you about Spiritism, because I know that you mock me in this regard, but if I don't often respond, *it's because they do not want it.* . . . You are going to say, *but why don't you tell him* [Marandon] *why you took the little girl? . . . Because I am possessed [obsédé]; the spirit that possesses me [mon obsesseur] is stronger than me,* or rather *than my mind;* and a Spiritist told me it is a suffering *soul*, and that my family is the cause of it; they must be delivered through prayers, and afterwards he will protect us.[50]

Fiquet then told a story about her father, who had suffered from the effects of somnambulism. In his sleep, or, as she claimed, under the influence of the malevolent spirit, her father had thrown himself out a third-floor window and been severely injured. It was not illogical for the woman to connect these ideas, since Spiritism, somnambulism, and hypnosis would later be seen as manifestations of the same phenomenon. As M. Brady Brower has noted, in *Unruly Spirits*, "The [Spiritist] medium exhibited the same symptoms of involuntarism, automatism, and disaggregation that had been observed in the somnambulant state produced by hypnosis."[51]

Fiquet's beliefs were essentially syncretic, and she happily blended elements of Catholicism, Protestantism, and Spiritism into her intellectual framework. Spiritism was a fundamentally modern belief system that emerged in the nineteenth century alongside the serious scientific study of hypnotism and somnambulism. Indeed, it was condemned by the Catholic Church as a subversive and radical current of thought. As a progressive invention with absolute freedom to define its own dogma, Spiritism crossed boundaries of class and gender, and it appealed particularly to women as a ritual that gave voice and hope to the oppressed, blurred gender boundaries (men could be reincarnated as women), and allowed people to imagine a better world than the one in which they struggled to exist. As a "deviant discourse," it was also easily classified within the framework of hysteria or madness by contemporary psychiatry.[52]

As Fiquet explained in her letter, her father recovered from his fall but afterward became a restless wanderer. Fiquet saw her troubles as emanating from his tendency toward automatism: *"In our family, I was the one destined to inherit this obsession."* She continued, "Please excuse me for allowing myself to write to you at such length on this subject, *but they are forcing me, I would not have said anything.* This is why I like cemeteries. *It is only in sad and lonely places that they listen to you."* Marandon said the investigating magistrate in Dijon was intrigued by this letter, concerned that this episode of hearing the dead talk revealed a hereditary mental disturbance, which potentially constituted a legitimate defense. Marandon was skeptical about the story, however: "Ordinarily, the criminal madman [*aliéné*] does not disclose his delusions, and he especially does not seek out similar ones, nor does he claim that his case has any precedent." Marandon saw Fiquet instead as a master of protean self-reinvention, of "simulation of the first order," pointing out the flagrant contradiction between her claim to be silenced by the possessing spirit and the telling and retelling of her story.[53]

In a second of the femme Fiquet's letters cited by Marandon and addressed to him, she wrote, "The reason for your visit was [to find out if] it was the spirit who had told me to abduct the little girl, my reply is *yes*. . . . If I went to the cemetery, to the grave of the two little children, it is because I was guided by the spirit that they had belonged to me in another existence."[54] The interconnecting stories that emerged in Fiquet's narrative—of child loss and child killing, poisoning, abortions, infanticides, cemeteries, spirits and souls, religiosity, the sacred, the maternal instinct, and the persistent preoccupation with medical scenes—point to a complex story of unresolved trauma and to a compulsion to repeat, within the context of a life as an unremarkable, impoverished working woman. Layers of evidence are there in the dossier, but Marie-Françoise Fiquet's intimate experiences were understood by her observers to be symptoms of an inherited bad character rather than the deep, driving elements in her life.

Marandon made an emphatic case, but he did not quite succeed in his intention of showing that beneath the simulation of spirit possession lurked a perfectly lucid, cold-blooded murderer trying to cover her tracks. Marandon even saw this flaw in his own argument and, remaining puzzled by the lack of motive, conceded finally that there must have been some underlying disturbance in his patient's character: "The *femme* Fiquet's entire life, as bizarre as it is villainous, her strange tendencies, her mania for frequenting hospitals to fool doctors and indulge herself, her passion for medical things including medicines, her religious machinations and many other things, everything about her points to an unbalanced nature, deprived of good judgment, an unreliable character, lacking perseverance and tenacity in her resolutions, as are proved by her contradictions even in this trial in which her very life is on the line."[55]

Although Marandon considered Fiquet's "possession" to be a simulation, her statements also conveyed an intense feeling of loss of control, of being a stranger to herself. She seemed to explain what in French would subsequently be theorized in the early twentieth century as the *acte gratuit*, a motiveless crime committed only for its own sake or on impulse. Downing argues that the classic *acte gratuit*, such as that described in Gide's *Les Caves du Vatican* (1914), where a man kills another for no other reason than feeling "the necessity to cede to impulse," is in modern culture typically viewed as a masculine act; this theme of being pushed to violence by an irresistible urge but for no clear reason also recurs in Albert Camus's novel, *L'Étranger* (1942).[56]

These were particularly modern perspectives on murder: Rather than through the religious framework of evil or the concept of psychological trauma, the inexplicable "impulse" in Fiquet's case was explained by her as originating in either a malevolent possessing spirit or the deranging effects of drugs. These were Fiquet's ways of making sense of her own actions, but they remained incomprehensible to her observers.

This drive to act, central to trauma, would be theorized soon after the Fiquet affair by Jean-Martin Charcot through his observations of hysterics under hypnosis. Charcot was head of a clinic at the Salpêtrière, the large women's public asylum in Paris, and in the 1880s was making his reputation as a theorist of the disease of hysteria, which he aimed to establish as a new and nosologically robust category.[57] Charcot's now-famous "Tuesday lessons" at the Salpêtrière, published from 1888 to 1894, were semipublic events that dramatically staged his clinic and were attended by many fashionable figures from the Parisian beau monde.[58] As Ruth Leys demonstrates in her study of the history of trauma,

> It is well known that the rise of trauma theory was associated from the start with hypnosis. Hypnosis, or hypnotic suggestion, was the means by which Charcot legitimated the concept of trauma by proposing that the hysterical crises that he suggestively induced in his patients were reproductions of traumatic scenes. What is less well understood is that hypnosis was not just an instrument of research and treatment but played a major theoretical role in the conceptualization of trauma. This is because the tendency of hypnotized persons to imitate or repeat whatever they were told to say or do provided a basic model for the traumatic experience. Trauma was defined as a situation of dissociation or "absence" from the self in which the victim unconsciously imitated, or identified with, the aggressor or traumatic scene in a condition that was likened to a state of heightened suggestibility or hypnotic trance. Trauma was therefore understood as an experience of hypnotic imitation or identification—what I call *mimesis*—an experience that, because it appeared to shatter the victim's cognitive-perceptual capacities, made the traumatic scene unavailable for a certain kind of recollection.

In her expression of a feeling of "possession," Fiquet was drawing on older explanatory frameworks that dated to the ancien régime and which found new expression in the nineteenth century. However, she also clearly articulated this sense of being absent from herself, as though hypnotized, the same phenomenon observed by Charcot. There is a connection between the ideas of demonic possession and sorcery, with the former being unwitting and the latter a conscious choice. As Thibaut Maus de Rolley has shown in the case of sorcery in seventeenth-century France,

> Any person deemed to be possessed was considered a victim of the devil, and who needed to be rescued, unlike witches and sorcerers, who needed to be exterminated. . . . Witches were bound to the devil by a formal pact. In exchange for this allegiance, they were given the power to perform a variety of evil deeds (*maleficia*): poisoning, infliction of disease, curses, killing newborn babies, destroying crops and livestock, unleashing storms and so on. Through their pact, they also joined a vast conspiracy whose ultimate goal was the ruin of the Church and the State. . . . The possessed woman, unless she later became a witch, had not made a pact with the devil and was not practicing evil spells. She was not a criminal.[59]

The possessed were not considered entirely innocent, since possession was thought to be a punishment for sin and because demons could only enter morally and spiritually weak bodies. However, a possessed woman (as victim of the devil) would have been subject to exorcism rather than a trial.[60] Structurally speaking, the same dilemma faced those who were to judge the femme Fiquet's crime. Was she acting under the influence of something she could not control, or were her actions chosen? At the end of the investigation, the femme Fiquet was found to be guilty and conscious of her actions, although it was admitted that she had exhibited some loss of control and therefore responsibility: Her mental strangeness and her morphine addiction meant it was possible she was not entirely conscious of her decisions. However, the accusations of poisoning, infanticide, and fraud suggested a pathological type of personal agency that necessitated her removal from society.

Marandon therefore cautiously recommended the recognition of these attenuating circumstances, not based on any conclusive medical symptom or even clear evidence but on his intuitions: "It is no less true that this affair remains a mysterious one, shrouded in darkness that cannot be explained by either morphinomania, or nervous madness. If the motive was not due to mental illness, it is not any less unknown and here there is a serious gap in the investigation that ought to make the expert circumspect in his conclusions when they may well lead to a death penalty."[61]

Marandon did offer, as an afterthought, a tentative theory as to what might have happened that day. Had Henriette been accidentally or deliberately sedated, perhaps to keep her quiet, and later drowned by Fiquet? "It seems to me from the examination of the prosecution case and Henriette's autopsy that she had been asleep for most of the day and drowned in a narcotic stupor between ten and eleven o'clock in the evening."[62] This theory fitted the pattern of behavior Fiquet had shown, that of administering noxious medicines to vulnerable people. Other than this theory, Marandon was frustrated not to find a convincing explanation that matched any known medical framework.

The Blanche Report

Marandon's report was initially considered sufficient evidence for the trial to go ahead. Proceedings were due to begin at the Dijon assizes court on 1 December 1882, but at the opening hearing of the *acte d'accusation* (indictment), the Fiquet couple's defense lawyers objected that they had not been informed of the charge of premeditation before the first reading. They requested more time both to prepare an adequate defense and for a second medical examination to be carried out.[63] The président of the court subsequently invited the Parisian hysteria expert, Charcot, to undertake the second medical examination.[64]

As we have just seen, Charcot's early work on hypnosis had been mentioned in Marandon's report as part of the body of published medical knowledge to which Fiquet would have had access in the fabrication of her nervous illnesses.[65] It is perhaps for this reason that the neurologist was called on as an expert. Charcot was not, however, primarily a medico-legist, which may be why he declined the brief—officially saying he was too busy to take the case. Instead, the dossier was passed on to another Parisian alienist, Dr. Émile Blanche. As part of a small group of elite medico-legists working in Paris at this time, Blanche came from a notable family (his son was the society painter Jacques-Émile Blanche; his father was also a celebrated alienist) and was famous enough to be considered by Dr. René Semelaigne, chronicler of the history of French alienist medicine, as one of the foremost pioneers of the discipline.[66] Émile Blanche was known as an expert who had testified in many of the most serious criminal cases of the era.[67]

Émile Blanche's father, Esprit Blanche, had established a private clinic (a *maison de santé*) at Passy, in the sixteenth district of Paris, in the mid-nineteenth century. The management of the clinic passed from father to son and was founded in the contemporary tradition of humanitarian alienism. It thus provided a homelike therapeutic environment, called the *vie de famille* method, where inmates could be gently brought back to reason through the use of "moral treatments," or talking therapies.[68] The clinic welcomed troubled and sometimes famous private clients, including the poet Gérard de Nerval and Théo van Gogh, the brother of Vincent; it is also where the syphilitic Guy de Maupassant ended his days in the 1890s.

Émile Blanche was therefore a respected expert whose view on Marie-Françoise Fiquet would be given significant weight in proceedings. In December 1882, the femme Fiquet was transferred from Dijon to the Saint-Lazare women's prison and infirmary in Paris. Dr. Blanche made several visits to observe and interview her before she returned to prison in Dijon in February 1883. Blanche's report is dated 4 February 1883 and was returned just one month before the trial began.

Dr. Blanche confirmed Marandon's conclusions but focused less on the theoretical details of "morphinomania" and more on the question of simulation. After attentively reading all the documentation relating to the case dossier—interrogations, witness statements, expert reports, letters, and the legal text of the indictment—Blanche concluded there were no prior signs of "mental alienation" in Fiquet's case. However, she told the doctor that as a fifteen-year-old she had been placed in the Salpêtrière asylum, under the name "Schneider," by a group of itinerant street performers with whom she was traveling through Paris. Blanche had this claim checked against the institutional records and found it to be false. This initial deception made him suspicious of Fiquet's other claims, such as her description of her father's somnambulism and other "alleged illnesses" that Blanche considered to be "either simulated or exaggerated."[69]

Blanche was also skeptical about the extent of Fiquet's dependency on morphine: "The accused woman did not present the characteristic symptoms of morphine intoxication either." Blanche assessed that the woman's intellectual faculties would only have been affected fleetingly by morphine, if at all. He also maintained that, had Fiquet really acted in a state of delusion, "she would have recognized the unconscious act that she had committed, and would have expressed her surprise" when returning to consciousness. The doctor pondered whether Fiquet had found herself under the spell of "an irresistible impulse" but concluded that she had not, because she had not reacted in bewilderment in front of her daughter when she realized what she had done.[70] Instead, she had constructed a web of lies to cover up her actions.

In addition to his regular visits to interview his patient, Dr. Blanche received letters from Marie-Françoise Fiquet. In his attempt to establish the truth of her mental state and moral responsibility, Blanche reproduced a *récit*, a story or narrative, related to him by his patient and charge, which took up three pages of the report. Blanche argued that Fiquet's claimed amnesia, as recounted in her narrative, was deceptive because it was selective: She clearly remembered some details of the day and conveniently had no memory of others. He also disbelieved her description of the effects of morphine: "She absolutely denied that she had caused [Henriette's] death, and claimed that, as a result of her hardened morphine abuse, it often happened that she wasn't aware of what she was doing."[71]

At the time of her arrest, Fiquet appeared to be preoccupied with her own guilt, believing a spirit guide had destined her for the scaffold: "I am accused of kidnapping a child, and worse than that, of murder; not of molestation, the child was untouched. I was arrested in June, I wanted to be condemned." The femme Fiquet then described taking Henriette from school back to her home. When the abduction happened, Fiquet insisted, "I was very ill that day, because I didn't have my syringe, I had drunk some morphine that morning, just like the previous evening, I didn't know what I was doing."[72]

By the time Blanche observed her, Fiquet had gone over her story several times, for the investigation and for other doctors. Elements of the account had stabilized, and Fiquet tried to present Henriette's death as a case of accidental poisoning, not drowning:

After dinner, I went to lie down; the little girl played with the dog, with some ribbons, and with my daughter's doll. In the afternoon, when I was in my bed, the child approached and took from the side table the bowl in which there was still some morphine potion; as it is very bitter, I had added a lot of sugar; she drank what was left in the bowl, there was still a lot of morphine in the bowl; she sat on a chair and fell asleep. So, I got up and laid her on the bed. I hadn't noticed when she took the bowl; I thought of it when I saw her asleep, I looked in the empty bowl, I hadn't seen her take it. She became very red, I put cold compresses on her forehead; she was already unconscious; . . . she was foaming at the mouth. Then my husband arrived home, I was crying, I was screaming, then he said to me, "What is this child doing here?" So, I said to him, "It's a little girl I brought home." Then he said to me, "But the child is dying!" He told me to go to the police; I was in a state! I didn't want to; the little girl died after three quarters of an hour; then he said to me, "This evening I will take her out into the street, someone will find her and take her home." . . . The evening came, my husband carried her away, he placed her at the edge of the canal, with her head in the water, as though she had fallen there accidentally.[73]

Despite Fiquet's insistence that this was her first confession, Blanche pointed out that in earlier statements she had told the same story but with varying features; for example, she had previously talked of giving the morphine solution to Henriette directly herself. According to the witness statements previously examined, Louise Fiquet had seen the little girl alive at lunchtime but did not see her again in the afternoon or evening. Pierre Fiquet insisted through all his testimonies that he had never seen the girl alive. However, the autopsy report found the cause of death to be drowning, and witnesses from the canal side that night had reported seeing a child walking with a woman. It is also implausible that the femme Fiquet could have carried Henriette for thirty to forty minutes, the time it would have taken to walk to the canal. The facts of what happened remain something of a mystery.

Throughout the narrative presented to Blanche, Fiquet oscillated between denial and culpability, remembering and forgetting. Her need to achieve oblivion—manifested in her dependency on morphine (to forget or remove physical and psychological pain)—was reiterated when she recounted using chloroform in response to the shock (as she claimed) of finding the little girl dead: "I was so sick that, to prevent my emotional crises, I took chloroform, which overcame me; I could not move anymore."[74] Fiquet used the French verb *accabler* to describe the effect of the chloroform, which carries multiple connotations: to be floored, crushed, or overcome but also to be accused; to be hit by a piece of damning evidence.[75] She was literally knocked out by the chloroform but was also perhaps, possibly at this moment and certainly at other moments, overcome with emotion when contemplating the gravity of her actions.

The same letter later contained a confused string of assertions that revealed a mind troubled by the need to forget her misdeed. Immediately following Henriette's death, Fiquet claimed to have spent the night reading, distracting herself from the events of the day: "I did not think about what had just happened to me."[76] Fiquet said that, although she hid things from herself, she did not conceal them from others: "I did not hide away from what I had done."[77] It was for this reason that she had been quickly discovered.

By the time she was arrested, the state of denial and oblivion had taken over. She said, "They came to arrest me; I had not been out, I didn't think about what had happened the day before, I had completely forgotten it. . . . I didn't remember anything, I denied everything." Fiquet consistently presented the events of Henriette's death as something that had happened to her rather than something she had done to a child. This added weight to her claim that she had acted on an irresistible impulse, one that made her a stranger to herself. Oblivion was a distancing mechanism. Fiquet tended to use imprecise formulations to describe her pain, such as "sick" or "very sick," being "in a state," and the verb *suffer* to describe her underlying state.

Blanche described her as an attention-seeking, capricious hysteric, whom the doctors ignored like a child having a tantrum: "She lets out screams, she twists her arms. . . . We let her cry without seeming to bother with her, and she quiets down."[78]

Fiquet claimed to be unable to resist external forces pushing her to kill, and other murderers have described their actions in similar terms. For example, those criminals invited by criminologist Lacassagne to make a written account of their actions also foregrounded the chaotic experience of contradictory internal drives. In 1905, Jean-Marie Bladier, a young seminarian who decapitated his best friend and was committed to a psychiatric asylum for life, outlined in his letters and autobiographical writings the intense conflict he felt between his murderous urges (described as an irresistible *passion*) and his moral sense of right and wrong.[79] According to Lacassagne, who studied Bladier's writing closely, the "criminal gesture" was often preceded by a period of meditation, or rumination, from which sprung the intellectual—and, arguably, libidinal—impulse to act.[80]

Blanche considered Fiquet's fickle and hazy memory to be a simulation and a cover for her premeditated actions. He suggested in his report that the episode with the twin babies might, too, have been a simulation: "She experienced periods of vagueness during which she had bizarre thoughts, such as taking an unknown child in the road, or to falsely announce to her husband that she had given birth to twin babies, or to make false declarations to appropriate these twins, and buying medical textbooks that she did not need."[81]

Fiquet's references to having an idée fixe for stealing children, and her obsession with midwifery, suggest she experienced an unresolved and paradoxical desire to nurture coexistent with a violent capacity to destroy children. This behavior is a classic example of perversion, as understood in psychoanalytical terms, in which the sexual instinct is redirected toward destruction instead of reproduction.[82] Yet Blanche, like Marandon before him, still struggled to understand what drove Fiquet because such connections were not yet being commonly made in criminal psychology. But Blanche's reference to Fiquet's acquisition of medical textbooks suggests a disappointed ambition that plausibly formed part of a wider frustration and desperation to make her mark on the world.

In the second *récit* given to Blanche, the femme Fiquet admitted that she went with her husband as far as the place Saint-Jean, halfway along the route to the canal, but claimed that he went on alone to the canal to leave the girl's body there. Two eyewitnesses saw a woman and a child at the canal side that night, so this seemed to be another fabrication. Fiquet continued her story and said more about this idée fixe, or obsession, with acquiring children. She spoke of it as an affliction:

> I only remembered these facts one day at the mental asylum, I had never yet said anything about it, I did not want to defend myself; I wanted to be condemned to death. My lawyer pleaded that I was insane; I am not insane, I am sick; he took me for a madwoman because he is a great believer, a devout Catholic, and because I am a Spiritist. Why would I want to be condemned to death? But is this a life, to always suffer and to have an *idée fixe* to abduct children, to bring them back to the house? I never wanted to harm any children.

The second part of Blanche's report integrated into his narrative Fiquet's direct words, taken from his final interviews with the accused woman. Her words are reproduced in italics. During their conversations, Fiquet apparently displayed psychiatric and spiritual disturbances:

> She attached a paper cross to the wall near her bed to keep the devil away, because they tell her *that only the devil could torment her like that. They cast spells on her, like in Dijon.* . . . She begs me not to go to so much trouble for her, not to come so often. *The more treatment I receive, the sicker I will be; this is not an illness that doctors can cure, it is a test; the medium in Besançon would have cured me. I was already arrested for arson in a previous life, and I already died in prison. I do not wish to be tormented in this way. I will no longer respond, they are all crazy, these people! I have accepted the indictment, I have nothing to add; this must end; I wanted to be condemned, because there are times when I do things without realizing, where I feel obliged to do what comes into my mind, what is suggested to me. You can see that I have been accused of murder, when it is my husband who is guilty and who got me into this mess.* . . .
>
> *I was sent here to be driven mad.* . . . *It has been planned out, a plot hatched against me. They mock my suffering; they say that I have marks on my back that look like those of a convict;* . . . *I know very well that I am not mad; you can't pretend to be crazy, you can't fool the doctors. I do not wish to return to Dijon, I want to be judged in Paris; there [in Dijon], they are under the influence of my obsessor.*[83]

I have translated literally the French word *obsesseur* used by Fiquet; it does not appear in French or English dictionaries, but it was used in specialist writing about Spiritism. It refers to the mind (of the *obsédé*) being taken over by a malign influence (that of the *obsesseur*). Fiquet clearly articulated in these letters, again, the urge she felt as an obligation to act imposed on her by this external force.

After his investigation, Blanche did not believe he was able to reveal any-thing new about the case: "In terms of information, she practically only repeated to me what she had already said in her interrogations; in reality, she did not add anything new. These conversations, and her letters, always revolved around her moral and physical pain and suffering, the inevitabil-ity of her fate, the influence of spirits on her actions, and her moments of oblivion; she just placed a greater emphasis on her spiritist practices. In her behavior, simulation played an important role."[84]

Blanche described his patient simulating visions, refusing food, experienc-ing weakness and memory loss—although he conceded that her dramatic ter-rors might have been at least partly genuine, because "the *femme* Fiquet must really be very tormented by her predicament." As for her claim to be guided by spirits, Blanche declined to comment on the doctrine but was skeptical: "It is impossible for me to admit that her own will was overridden by what she calls 'the will of her obsessor.'"[85]

Blanche's comments on Fiquet's claim to be controlled by spirits reflected the era in which he was writing. The discipline of psychical research that would later become part of scientific psychology was a nascent field in the later nineteenth century. It was also treated with skepticism by established alienists and other specialists (such as neurologists). Although Spiritism had become a popular international movement from the early 1850s, and it clearly influenced Fiquet in her understanding of her own mental pro-cesses, psychical phenomena did not become a serious topic of medical and psychological research until the 1880s, with organizations such as the Insti-tut Général Psychologique representing researchers not being established until 1900.[86] This field of research was significant because it contributed to emergent psychological ideas of a "decentered and fragmented subject."[87] It pointed toward the conceptualization of the unconscious in the twentieth century by thinkers such as Pierre Janet, Sigmund Freud, and Carl Jung.[88] And it would be, above all, psychoanalysis that would lay the groundwork for psychodynamic theories of trauma and perversion.

Marie-Françoise Fiquet communicated the idea that she was driven by unconscious forces or spirits. As noted, ideas of unconscious motivation were only just beginning to be explored in the 1880s, when thinkers such as Charles Richet and Pierre Janet began to challenge the idea that the mind could be considered unified and self-identical.[89] The same process of questioning whether it was possible to know oneself and to always act rationally was also being applied to the judicial process. The Spiritist beliefs Fiquet exhibited were popular among women and would, according to Brady Brower, "con-tinue to bear strong associations with middle- and lower-middle class religiosity."[90] If we mobilize a psychodynamic interpretive framework, Fiquet's desire to communicate with the dead, just as she harmed and killed innocent people, points to an unconscious psychological repetition compulsion.

The medical assessment was conclusive in its findings that the femme Fiquet was neither insane nor driven out of her mind by morphine; neither was she a hypochondriac. Blanche also concluded that on 29 June 1882, she was not unaware of what she was doing, nor did she "cede to a morbid and irresistible impulse," despite her claims to the contrary. Blanche's most trenchant point is that Fiquet's claimed state of confusion conflicted with the apparent lucidity with which she recalled the events of that day—an "elective amnesia" that applied only to her incriminating actions. He declared that she could be considered criminally responsible but that she suffered from a type of mental agitation, common to "simulators," that ought to be considered a mitigating factor.[91] Blanche and Marandon were, in the end, sympathetic to the possibility that Fiquet was in some distress and experienced some remorse and that Henriette's death could have been at least partly accidental, even if it had been the result of the femme Fiquet's bizarre behavior.

Most importantly, Fiquet's inveterate morphine use, although cast as a "passion," did not mitigate Fiquet's actions—even though she clearly articulated her distress, pains, losses, and addictions. Blanche and Marandon were not convinced that Marie-Françoise Fiquet had taken as much morphine as she claimed, nor that she was ever in a state of extreme intoxication; it followed, therefore, that withdrawal could not have been considered a major problem. Even if Fiquet had been in withdrawal, they concluded, the resultant behavior would have likely been "acts of dementia or rage" rather than coolly premeditated murder.[92]

In his conclusions, Blanche admitted that Fiquet's arms were covered in needle marks—to the modern observer, perhaps, the sure sign of addiction and hardened habitual use—but still insisted this was no evidence of quantity of use, and therefore of effect. After all, an addict does not a murderer make. "Although we can believe that she used this substance to calm her headaches, as she claims, and to procure 'a state of wellbeing,' we have never observed in her the disorders that are produced by a true intoxication."[93] The net result of both doctors' conclusions was that Fiquet's morphine addiction was sidelined as an explanatory factor in the trial that followed. On the question of her psychiatric disturbance, the principal presenting symptoms of "simulation" and the need to cede to irresistible impulse were read as evidence of the *absence* of illness. Blanche and Marandon were unable, in 1882–83, to conceive of simulation itself as part of a diagnostic picture of the wide-ranging factitious disorder that in retrospect it seems to have been.

The Troppmann Affair and the Femme des Batignolles

The Troppmann Affair

Many features of the Fiquet affair can be compared with criminal cases that occurred in the decades preceding and following it. Such cases highlight contemporary reactions to what were considered the dangerous and deviant behaviors of working-class men and women. The moralizing tone of the press accounts of these cases served the purpose of warning the ruling classes of the dangers posed by the masses. The working classes were often seen as a release valve for humanity's destructive sexual and violent urges, elsewhere contained by civilizing processes; cases where this process went awry illustrated starkly what could happen when those drives were turned back onto innocent people rather than expelled.[1] Personal ambition, high intelligence, and the ruthless drive for recognition and status were all considered suspicious and dangerous traits. The purpose of this interlude is to show that, collectively, these cases were indicative of a profound but unfulfilled need for security, status, agency, and connection in the lives of the new urban working classes, during a period of social change driven by urbanization, modernization, and the associated psychological alienation it brought. I focus on two cases: that of Jean-Baptiste Troppmann, who in 1869 murdered an entire family near Paris, apparently for money, and that of the abortionist Constance Thomas, popularly known as the femme des Batignolles, who was convicted in 1891.

The Troppmann affair was a contemporary parallel to the Fiquet affair; as "one of the greatest *faits divers* of the nineteenth century," it influenced the press reporting of later murder cases across France.[2] Troppmann was a migrant worker from Alsace who was resourceful, ruthless, and ambitious. Just a decade before Marie-Françoise Fiquet killed Henriette Barbey, Troppmann had been found guilty of murdering the Kinck family at Pantin, an industrial, distant suburb of Paris. The mother of the family, who was six months pregnant, and the bodies of her five youngest children were found first. The body of Gustave, her eldest son, was found in a nearby spot three days later. Finally, Troppmann admitted having poisoned the father, Jean Kinck, using prussic acid (hydrogen cyanide). His body was found hidden in some local woodland in November, two months after the others.[3]

Troppmann appealed for clemency against the death penalty but lost; he was guillotined in 1870. The exceptional features of the case were the brutality of the murders (the bodies were gratuitously mutilated) and the lack of motive. Why would anyone want to kill a whole family? It would come to be known as "Le crime de Pantin," like the later murder of Henriette Barbey would be called "Le crime de Dijon," and the case was taken up enthusiastically by the emergent large-distribution press of the era.

Troppmann was, according to French historian Michelle Perrot, a "sensational criminal event" that would provoke lively discussion in the press and contribute to the commercial success of penny publications such as *Le Petit Journal*, which targeted new working-class consumers. The story captured the imagination of the public who were drawn to the tidbits of information provided via the daily *fait divers* rubric. Under the Second Empire, the police had developed investigative technologies that enabled them to gather evidence in novel ways. The reporting of these procedures made for interesting copy and created suspense for readers. During the Troppmann investigation, for example, the forensic experts detected traces of prussic acid in Jean Kinck's intestines, proving he had been poisoned.[4] Similarly, the forensic experts in the Fiquet case dissected Henriette Barbey's stomach but found no trace of morphine, compounding the mystery surrounding the murder.

In both cases the working-class protagonists were presented according to commonly understood stereotypes. The subaltern classes were viewed as both dangerous, typified in the figures of Fiquet, Troppmann, and other killers, and incarnating an ideal of virtue. Perrot has pointed out the emphasis in the press on the bravery of a man named Hauguel who apprehended Troppmann and "was celebrated as the incarnation of the people, serving the cause of justice."[5] Similarly, Marie-Françoise Fiquet's daughter, Louise; the factory workers; and the family's neighbors were all cast in the early press reports in Dijon as "good" working people who had helped eject the bad apples from their own communities. The concept of "honest" or "decent" working folk was pervasive and represented people trying their best to do right, even though sometimes, through forced error, they fell from the path of virtue.

One of the most famous examples of this type of representation is the character of Fantine in Victor Hugo's Les Misérables (1862), who is abandoned by her feckless lover and devotes herself selflessly to caring for their young daughter, Cosette.[6] Women like Fiquet were considered beyond redemption in their calculated selfishness and shameless exploitation of others. She represented a different working-class stereotype—that of women of the "dangerous classes" whose moral limitations and tendency to irresponsibility was the direct cause of their own misery and extreme poverty.

The Kincks were presented as having achieved success through hard work and virtuous devotion to their family unit. As Perrot notes, "The city council raised funds to erect a monument in the city cemetery to the family, who had become a symbol of goodness destroyed by crime."[7] Similarly, in the Fiquet case, the Barbeys were consistently presented as decent and honest folk, though this was to a certain extent a fantasy. Evidence to the contrary would emerge in later press reports, which showed that Mr. Barbey was a chronic alcoholic; he would also be convicted a few years later of molesting his young niece.[8] The reality, therefore, was that the Barbey family was as dysfunctional and troubled by addiction and dysregulated behavior as the Fiquet family and so many others were.

In contrast to the victims, the procureur insisted on Troppmann's dark, brooding, angry personality and on his greed. He was directly motivated by the personal humiliation he felt as a member of the lower classes; Fiquet's insistently attention-seeking behavior suggested that she also believed she was special, different from her peers and deserving of recognition. Troppmann was a hardworking and gifted mechanic and inventor who had asked Jean Kinck to finance one of his inventions. He was also a fantasist and a dreamer who devoured racy and popular romans-feuilletons (serial novels) and claimed as an inspiration Eugène Sue's Le Juif errant, in which a character called Rodin kills a rich family to lay claim to their millions. The press suspected that the highly suggestible Troppmann had been perverted by unhealthy reading habits.[9]

Historical records that provide rich material for micro investigations often come into existence because ordinary people refuse to accept or submit to their ordinariness; in their struggle to rise above it, they occasionally ran into trouble with the law. Zemon Davis has argued that this was a key motivation in the case of Martin Guerre: "Martin dreamed of life beyond the confines of millet, of tileworks, properties, and marriages."[10] This idea of the "life beyond" is also a connecting thread in the cases of Troppmann and Fiquet. In the late 1890s, the criminals encouraged by Professor Alexandre Lacassagne in Lyon to write their life stories would also be marked with this concern to communicate their "need to be recognized not as vulgar criminals but as exceptional individuals."[11] Lacassagne wanted to understand what motivated proletarian criminal behavior and studied their writings to this end. Even the suspected serial killer of women Henri Vidal wrote a letter (before being shipped to the penal colony in Guyana, in 1902) explaining that Lacassagne was the only man who had ever really understood him and who had seen into his wounded soul.[12]

The distinction between the virtuous and the dangerous working classes was reflected, also, in the opposing concepts of "the people," represented by the heroes who helped to bring criminals to justice, and "the crowd" that sought to mete out extrajudicial justice and had to be contained. Both were powerful social forces that needed to be carefully calibrated. In 1870, Charles Hugo wrote in *Le Rappel*, "For the people is magnanimous, and this crowd is ferocious."[13] The crowd was an emotional, punitive mob, but the virtuous "people" were dispassionate, just, and judicious. This distinction between the masses as good and the crowds they formed as potentially dangerous was mirrored in the view of women as either trustworthy or dangerous, depending on the spaces they inhabited. As Elissa Gelfand has noted, "Notions of a 'dangerous' or 'suspect' woman centered on her family role. . . . Thus widows, orphans, and vagabond and exiled women, by their rootless sexual status, were the most vulnerable to accusation and the most severely punished. Such women threatened the model of family sexual stability that Rousseau and other eighteenth-century philosophers developed into paradigms of social utility and general welfare."[14]

Marie-Françoise Fiquet slipped between these two categories, which arguably made her even more dangerous. She was married, employed, and a mother. This meant that people instinctively trusted her—most significantly, Henriette Barbey trusted her. But Fiquet had also been a rootless wanderer, and stories about her sexual immorality were leveraged to categorize her as a member of the dangerous crowd, when all the while she was masquerading as a virtuous, "normal" working woman.

La Femme des Batignolles

Constance Thomas, the midwife and abortionist known as *la femme des Batignolles*, would be convicted in Paris alongside her accomplice Abelard Floury in 1891, eight years after the Fiquet affair. Thomas was sentenced to twelve years of hard labor; Floury received a lesser sentence for handling the money paid for the procedures. Thomas claimed to have performed illegal abortions on more than four thousand women, from all echelons of society. These included respectable married women, many of whom had acted with the full knowledge of their husbands.[15] Ryckère, in his discussion of criminal women, described Thomas's defense—that she was helping women who would otherwise endanger themselves by engaging in more hazardous practices—as "extraordinary," and Thomas was apprehended after her last client died in hospital after her abortion.[16]

There were striking parallels between the Thomas case and that of Marie-Françoise Fiquet. They both came from humble, rural origins and were thrown out of their respective family homes due to disreputable conduct. Thomas moved to the city with another girl who had also been driven out of her village for the same reason. The abortionist, too, was highly intelligent and had been, in the journalist Maurice Talmeyr's words, "hypnotized" by her country-doctor uncle's library of books, just as Fiquet had acquired and become obsessed with medical textbooks. Both women were willing to take risks and began their illicit activities at a young age, probably in their late teens. Thomas was considered a debauched, amoral, brazenly promiscuous thief. She appeared to show callous indifference toward the women she later "treated" but had, like Fiquet, been deeply affected by the loss of her first baby, a girl, whom she had nursed affectionately but who died at six months old.[17]

In an account of the Constance Thomas case and trial presented in a series of articles published in the republican literary periodical *Gil Blas* in 1891, Talmeyr insisted on the physiognomic evidence of evil, characterized in part by uncertain gender: "Constance Thomas is now forty-seven years old and her rough, weathered countenance is typical of the hideous types collected by anthropometrists. The deep wrinkles and veins drawn on her pudgy face seem to excrete all kinds of corruption, and she seems to breathe evil through the nostrils of her manly nose." Criminal women were paradoxically cast as naturally corrupt in their femininity but also evil because of the loss of that femininity. Gelfand has argued that both normality and deviance for women were rooted in the body: "The many nineteenth-century treatises on female criminality vary only in their terminology; all reaffirm—whether as 'perversion,' 'moral insanity,' or 'mental degeneration'—the noncognitive and 'natural' source of female deviance."[18]

In the front-page illustration for the *Gil Blas* report, Constance Thomas's and her co-accused Abelard Floury's faces look interchangeably rough and masculine, contrasted with the feminine, angelic, ghostly face of the dead woman who appears behind them, as if the pure and innocent victim of their determined schemes. These same physiognomic signs of corruption would be noted in the Fiquet trial, as we shall see in chapter 5.

Also apparent in the Constance Thomas case was the suggestion of a psychological repetition compulsion and the drive to carry out abortions on a massive scale: Thomas was meeting a demand, but she was not simply providing a service. She also seemed to gain secondary satisfaction from perfecting and controlling the procedure. To this end, she acted with a boldness that shocked her contemporaries. In his article on the Thomas case, René Le Mée has hypothesized that the root of Thomas's compulsive behavior lay in the specific trauma of losing a baby she had cherished: "Was the shock caused by this loss so great that it caused her to reject the child, to the extent that she felt she was doing a favor to the women who came to her for help—for this seems to have been her state of mind when she was 'operating' on them?"[19]

Talmeyr related that Constance Thomas theatrically passed out briefly every time she performed an abortion, at the specific moment of accomplishing the act. She took satisfaction in noting the cleanliness and efficiency of her procedures and the ritual departure of yet-to-be-born infants to the afterlife under her guidance.[20] We might infer that Thomas was not acting simply out of a desire to help women in difficult situations; she actively enjoyed the control she exercised over life and death and had a sadistic desire to keep doing it. Human motivations are complex, and apparently altruistic actions can be tinged with egotism.

Sadism as a clinical category had not yet been described: it would be first expounded in Richard von Krafft-Ebing's *Psychopathia Sexualis* in 1886. Medico-legists such as Dr. Albert Moll, who would publish a treatise on the topic in 1893, thought that for a crime to be considered truly sadistic, it needed to have an unambiguously sexual element—here, they were referring to male paraphilias that tipped over into accidental or deliberate killing.[21] Although Thomas and Fiquet did not fit the clinical profile of sexual sadism, there is a clear sense in both narratives of libidinal pleasure accrued to them through their actions. This pleasure taken in the satisfaction of a dark desire was articulated in their cases through the ideas of appetite and compulsion.

This idea of repetition and the link to satisfaction taken in killing links to the parallel accusation of poisoning in the Fiquet case. Poisoning could also be framed as a type of morbid craving or irresistible urge. Ernest Dupré, in a psychological study of poisoners published in 1909, insisted on this point: "These crimes, often committed serially and without motive, seem therefore to be a means of satisfying morbid appetites: a thirst for suffering and death."[22]

Both women were ominously obsessed with medical textbooks and procedures, just as Troppmann was inspired by the dramas of working-class people depicted in contemporary novels. The common thread in these three cases was the coexistence of high intelligence, curiosity, and autodidacticism. The three accused criminals were at least partly motivated by anger and wanting to settle old scores—whether financial disappointment, shattered dreams, or the arbitrary cruelty of infant mortality. Envy was also central to all three cases. Troppmann envied Kinck's success and fortune and tried to emulate it: his failure to do so drove him to kill the family. Perhaps Fiquet and Thomas also envied the pregnant women they "treated" and, having been powerless to prevent the loss of their own infants, wanted to control life and death. Fiquet's desire to become a midwife, and failure to access the profession legitimately, plausibly produced burning frustration and envy in her.

The Troppmann murders were shown in the end to have been motivated by money and personal ambition. Troppmann was also, perhaps not coincidentally, an unusual and compelling personality. Although he personified evil, he was reported to be handsome and clever, a gifted mechanic and inventor who believed he could make a fortune. Troppmann was admired for his debonaire elegance and studied, courteous demeanor in the courtroom. Although monstrous, he was also impressive and even beautiful. The affair therefore followed the tradition of the romanticization of the male murderer as a heroic, youthful rebel and an outlaw, indeed an artist.[23] Troppmann's sleek presentation contrasted starkly with the brutality of his crimes, and his exaggerated preening was also a red flag for the audience, who perceived him as abnormally feminine, almost feline in his movements, suggestive of sexual deviance.[24]

In the cases of Troppmann and Fiquet, the reporting of court proceedings scrutinized the defendants' physical presentation and the revelation of underlying criminality and perversion. They were cast as pathologically ambitious and self-serving personalities who used their ruthless ingenuity to further their own interests. Troppmann wanted to be a rich man and refused to accept his mediocre destiny; he killed the Kinck family as part of an elaborate plan to acquire their fortune. Marie-Françoise Fiquet sought to control her own life and affairs, as well as those of others who were weaker than her; she manipulated the people around her to this end.

Troppmann's defense attorney framed his ambition as a form of monomania, an idée fixe that clouded his moral judgment. His mechanical inventions were manifestations of this "delusional monomania" that allowed him to believe he could become rich and successful.[25] The respective motives of Fiquet and Troppmann were therefore obscure and psychologically complex.

The press coverage in both instances involved the laundering of this complexity and the flattening out of ambiguities to present a coherent narrative to a fascinated but alarmed public.

Perrot showed how Troppmann was transformed, via the press, from a *fait divers* into a *grande affaire*. Fiquet was not such a famous case across France, although it was a locally significant true crime story. It was mediatized on a small scale in recorded documents that offer insights into contemporary attitudes, beliefs, and medical views on female violence. Historian Karine Salomé has argued that the process of fictionalization in the press reporting was significant in the case of Troppmann. For Salomé, the press emphasized the singular brutality of the crimes and the horror of the public at Troppmann's ruthless machinations.[26] These peculiar features also contributed to public interest in the murder of Henriette Barbey: a child victim who was particularly shy and fearful, an unusually violent death via drowning or deliberate poisoning, and a manipulative perpetrator.

All three cases considered in this interlude were crimes that stood outside contemporary norms: The victims, modes of killing, apparently perverse motives that went beyond comprehensible intentionality, and casual attitudes exhibited by the defendants all pointed to them as exceptional events.[27] Some crimes were comprehensible; others defied logic and inspired terror. A drunken brawl that went too far or the murder of an unfaithful spouse by a jealous husband could be shocking but might be viewed as possible or even inevitable when people were pushed into an altered state or beyond what they could emotionally tolerate. A crime became an "affaire" when it led commentators to reflect more deeply on human nature or when it unsettled contemporary models of motivation, mind, and the social order.

CHAPTER 5

The Trial

The trial of Marie-Françoise and Pierre Fiquet
commenced at the Palais de Justice in Dijon at eight o'clock in the morning
on Monday, 5 March 1883, nine months after Henriette Barbey's body was
found. It would last for three consecutive days. The couple were represented
separately by two remarkable men, Étienne Metman, who had the unenvi-
able task of defending Marie-Françoise Fiquet, and Paul Cunisset, who represented her husband. Metman, who turned forty in 1883, had a reputation in
Dijon as the "advocate of the poor." He was a passionate man: a champion of
the poor who was politically conservative, devoutly Catholic, and something
of an intellectual.[1] He would go on to publish several books, including the
1892 philosophical study *Le pessimisme moderne*, and a lengthy 1914 architectural history, *L'Église Saint-Michel de Dijon*. There is a road named after
Étienne Metman in the newer suburb of Dijon, Chenôve.

Metman's assistant, Paul Cunisset, was in his early thirties; a keen hunts-
man and fisherman, he had served with distinction in the Franco-Prussian
War and was at the beginning of what would prove a glittering legal career.
Later the same year he would marry Claire Carnot, daughter of Marie
François Sadi Carnot, who from 1887 until his assassination (by an Italian
anarchist) in 1894 would be president of France. As Paul Cunisset-Carnot,
the lawyer would go on to become deputy mayor of Dijon, procureur de
la République, and président de la cour d'appel de Dijon, and he would

also publish several books.[2] Much less is known about the public prosecutor (*l'avocat-général*) Mairet, although both his and Metman's summing-up speeches would be singled out for rapturous praise in the press.[3]

Such was the local interest in the case that by seven o'clock an eager crowd had gathered outside the court buildings, keen to gain access to a hearing that, according to *La Démocratie Bourguignonne*, "for many months had greatly excited public opinion in Dijon." Inside the courtroom, additional benches had been installed to accommodate the expected audience, while guards were placed at the doors to keep out the peering crowds who had not managed to get seats inside.[4] Jury trials in the *cour d'assises* (criminal court) began with the public swearing in of each juror, followed by the reading aloud of the *acte d'accusation*: the indictment, or the case against the accused. The reading of the *acte* was far from a neutral summary. It could often be a long and partisan character assassination of the accused person that included any details the public prosecutor wished to highlight for the audience.[5] The Fiquet indictment was, by contrast, brief and factual:

> The *femme* Fiquet and her husband Fiquet are accused of: 1. having, on June 29, 1882, in Dijon, intentionally caused the death of Henriette Barbey, acted with premeditation in attacking the person of the aforementioned Henriette Barbey; 2. having, on the same day and at the same place, stolen a comb and earrings from Henriette Barbey.

Like the death of Henriette, the trial would receive extensive and detailed coverage in the regional press, and both were also briefly reported nationally. The trial was reported at length in the moderately left-wing *Démocratie Bourguignonne* and garnered the attention of the more conservative press, the *Bien Public*, the *Côte-d'Or*, the *Progrès de la Côte-d'Or*, and was summarized in the weekly edition of the *Catholique*. But the reports in these daily papers were based on the more detailed coverage of the court proceedings given in the *Démocratie Bourguignonne*, which I focus on here.[6]

As Berenson has observed, French courtrooms could be somewhat anarchic, and the président did not always have strong authority over the room:

> The conduct of the Cour d'assises itself created a theatrical atmosphere that helped make press accounts even more compelling. Defendants, attorneys, witnesses, and even the presiding judge himself were allowed long soliloquies that enabled them to appeal beyond the jury to public opinion at large. And in making their appeals, they were hindered by few legal or procedural constraints. . . . Extensive as the Président's powers were, they were far from absolute. He did not pos-

sess the right to discipline either counsel unless he could demonstrate that one or the other had created a "tumult" in the courtroom. But because the Cour d'assises was regularly in a state of tumult—few settings could be more explosive than a felony court in which defendant, attorneys, witnesses, and judge could say almost anything to almost anyone with impunity—it was impractical for a Président to attempt to discipline a lawyer, no matter how provocative.

Robert A. Nye has also argued that second- and thirdhand accounts of crime, such as those found in news reports and popular culture, are important because they define the "public consciousness of crime." Criminal trials therefore grant us a unique perspective on the historical time and place in which they occurred.[7] This concurs with Foucault's point that, in the press, murder is a "privileged event" at "the crossing point of history and crime."[8] The courtroom is an adversarial space in which conflicts are staged, and Dominique Kalifa has observed that the trial is a multilayered reconstitution of the crime, culminating in the great "paroxysm of representation that is the theatre of the assizes court." The function of the preceding investigation was, therefore, to "render the crime representable."[9]

French juries, which were always used in the assizes courts for criminal trials, at this point were entirely made up of male jurors. James M. Donovan has shown how the introduction of jury trials during the Revolution (in 1791) gave the ordinary people that composed them a voice independent of political authorities and a means of resisting the rigid and punitive directives of the Napoleonic Penal Code.[10] Juries tended to be lenient, and André Gide observed in 1913 that jurors seemed conflicted when trying to reconcile the demands of objective truth, the legal code, and natural justice.

The drama of trials stemmed from this power struggle between the various actors in the theater of the court. Lawyers, according to Edward Berenson, were powerful and capable of obstructing the progress of trials altogether. Furthermore, the power of the press went virtually unchecked, and, unlike in England, newspapers often leaked details about cases and defendants before trials took place. In addition, the press had a wide reach. Most French people could read by the late nineteenth century, and most of them would have seen daily papers in some format. Readers were typically entertained by the thrills of the *fait divers*, the blurring of fact and fiction, and the presentation of true crime stories alongside novels by famous writers.[11]

There were two social conflicts staged in the Fiquet trial. First, the femme Fiquet had to face her audience—prosecutors, onlookers, jury, and press—alone. Despite her advocate, she was physically and psychologically isolated.

Second, there was a clash between legal and medical knowledge. Fiquet's was not a crime of passion, a definition reserved for "normal" people driven temporarily to act with uncontrolled violence but without premeditation.[12] It was an inexplicable act of perversion.

The press reports of the trial blended layers of moralizing narrative, with the effect of underlining, in Foucault's terms, the murderer's "shameful gesture" while sidelining entirely Fiquet's explanation of how she had come to kill Henriette: Nineteenth-century newspapers were "conformist and moralistic. They taught a lesson. They carefully distinguished the glorious act of the soldier from the shameful act of the assassin."[13] The process of designating Fiquet as an exceptional criminal, who violated the cultural codes of femininity, which had already emerged in the press reporting of the case in the days following Henriette's death, extended through the trial reporting.

Even her defense attorney, Metman—sensing, perhaps, the lack of sympathy in the courtroom for his client—did not try to claim that Fiquet had not caused Henriette's death. He focused on the likelihood of undetected mental instability and the distant possibility of accidental killing. Metman neither relied on the deterministic, Lombrosian view of the born female criminal nor attempted to present his case in terms of social determinism; in other words, he did not argue that Fiquet's milieu, morphine abuse, and life experiences were instrumental factors in her crime.[14] The press trial reports revealed new details concerning Fiquet's character and past life as well as further evidence of the sexual double standard in relation to Pierre Fiquet's treatment. They also dramatized the courtroom narrative in important ways.

As Gayle K. Brunelle and Annette Finley-Croswhite observed in the later case of the mysterious political murder of the spy and gadabout Lætitia Toureaux, in 1930s Paris, the social judgment imposed (or not) on victims and perpetrators was heavily gendered where women stepped outside accepted behavioral norms: "Denizens of the bals musette, especially if they were young women, never came to good ends. Journalists implied that happy endings were reserved only for those who adhered to traditional values that were grounded in respectability, Christian values, and patriarchal authority."[15] Similarly, there would be no sympathy for the femme Fiquet. As her family members, neighbors, and doctors testified, she defied social norms and had brought trouble on herself.

The press reporting of the Fiquet trial emphasized the role of the crowd and the emotional engagement of the audience throughout the proceedings. Fiquet's appearance, posture, facial expressions, words, and gestures were heavily dramatized: In Le Droit Populaire, the journalist reported on "the singular physiognomy of the femme Fiquet . . . a strange creature suspected of having poisoned her husband and an old Spiritist woman whom she had lured to her home." Her "simulated" illness was on display for all to see, as Fiquet was transported into the courtroom on "a makeshift bed" because she was "supposedly" suffering from sciatica and was too weak to sit or stand.[16] Some reports in the national press even suggested Fiquet had recently given birth in prison.[17]

Investigations privileged certain types of respectable female witnesses: virtuous mothers, wives, fiancées. In journalistic reports, women tended to be depicted as "not belonging" in judicial procedures; they were typically ill at ease and diffident or crass and inappropriate—like the femme Fiquet. Those who appeared confident and to "own the room," as Fiquet was reported to have done at certain moments during the trial, were considered suspicious self-dramatizers. For example, Kalifa has cited a report that appeared in *Le Journal* on 4 November 1902 on the trial of the serial killer Henri Vidal, in which female witnesses expressed "a little vain satisfaction at the idea of playing a role in a sensational affair."[18]

Accordingly, even as she faced the possibility of condemnation to death, the femme Fiquet's demeanor in the courtroom was depicted in the press coverage as a self-dramatizing fraud. Reporters expressed skepticism about her alleged physical incapacity, and all the doctors who testified considered her to be an eccentric simulator, "a cunning, attention-seeking woman."[19] Fiquet's sharp mind, wit, and intelligence were all emphasized in contrast to her husband's imbecility. The *Démocratie Bourguignonne* noted how the accused woman captured the room, how her "gleaming, black eyes still seem to have the same intensity we noticed in her the first time."[20] The *Progrès* added a waspish comment on her looks: "She is far from beautiful, and it is difficult to understand, from her appearance, the [sexual] successes of her youth."[21] These physiognomic signs cast Fiquet as a "born criminal" whose physical traits revealed her pathological nature: She was cruel, ugly, indolent, and perverted.[22] Similarly, Fiquet's drug use and sexual behavior were presented as being driven by her pathological appetites rather than as survival strategies.

Pierre Fiquet, by contrast, appeared childlike and simple: "Pierre Fiquet sits in the dock; he has a calm demeanor but still has the same characteristically unintelligent look about him. He seems oblivious to the seriousness of the accusation and appears very composed."[23] This was even noted in the national press, with the *Figaro* commenting, "The *femme* Fiquet's husband, facing trial as her accomplice, is a type of semi-idiot."[24] The emphasis on his composed appearance connoted innocence and a peaceful conscience. The *Démocratie Bourguignonne* added, "He seems to have valiantly tolerated the eight months of precautionary detention that he has just completed; his attitude is calm; but nothing about him suggests he is intelligent."[25]

Paradoxically, despite the insistence on Fiquet's dangerous intellectual power and troubling physiognomy, her voice throughout the trial reporting was effaced. Her statements were reduced to pithy and cursory summaries, dismissed as irrational and incomprehensible. One report noted that, when interrogated, "the accused woman speaks with a very faint voice and the president is obliged to have her repeat her responses several times."[26] It would seem that she was too weak to speak clearly, although her physical state was not noted beyond the early descriptions of her being carried in on a bed, and her claims to illness were dismissed as simulations.

The reporters also rarely cited the direct explanations given by Marie-Françoise Fiquet in her own defense, relying on formulations such as "the accused denies this" or "the accused gives an unintelligible explanation."[27] Just as Fiquet was presented as hypersexualized, prostituting herself to all and sundry, she was also—paradoxically—virilized through assertions about her extensive intellectual capacities, domineering character, and capacity for violence. This amounted to a portrait of a highly atypical woman who defied codes of ideal and virtuous femininity and lacked humility. The newspapers reported little of what Fiquet *said* in her trial. Her own explanation—that she had been profoundly changed by the influence of morphine addiction, possessed by spirits, and acting on irresistible impulse—disappeared completely from the narrative.

Significant time was given over in the trial to the examination of Fiquet's antecedent character, specifically to the allegations of poisoning, her fraudulent attempts to practice midwifery and clandestine abortions, and her sexual morality: It seemed she was guilty of every imaginable gendered crime as well as the one for which she was standing trial. This evidence was drawn out through the interrogations of the femme Fiquet and her husband, as well as the witness testimonies, and was dramatized through descriptions of the audience reactions.

For the prosecution, Mairet began by questioning Fiquet on her life from childhood, her unrestrained sexual behavior, and her manipulation of religious authority figures to her financial advantage. He reported that when she arrived at Vonges (a commune in the Côte-d'Or administrative *département*, east of Dijon) with her family as a young woman, to work in the vineyards, "You left the most unfortunate memories in that place: your conduct was poor, and you were lazy."[28] Mairet went on to report a series of incidents involving Marie-Françoise Fiquet as a young woman, including getting pregnant at fifteen, being evicted from lodgings in Dijon in 1873 for bringing a soldier back to her room one night, and carrying out theft in Besançon in 1874. "The president has Monsieur Jouchou's [the alleged victim] declaration read out on the subject of this theft; it concludes by saying that the *femme* Fiquet was lazy, intemperate and lived an immoral life and appeared to be in full possession of her intellectual faculties."[29]

Fiquet denied everything, and Metman, in her defense, objected to these unsubstantiated allegations being leveraged as circumstantial evidence against his client. However, the président was entirely satisfied that the anecdotal evidence seemed to "corroborate the rumors of abortion" that had circulated around the unmarried Marie-Françoise Rémond (the femme Fiquet) during her teenage years.[30] Since undetected infanticide and clandestine abortion were relatively common during this period, the story would have been plausible to the people listening. The audience seemed unmoved by Fiquet's defense. Mairet kept them entertained and horrified, citing an occasion when Fiquet had asked a nurse in the asylum "how a person driven mad by morphine abuse would behave." The nurse had cannily replied, "She would be sad, thoughtful, and she would work hard." The next day, Fiquet conveniently became sad, thoughtful, and industrious. Mairet's sarcastic account was greeted with great "hilarity in the audience."[31]

During questioning about a theft, Fiquet claimed that she had stolen a man's watch because he had raped her. Mairet responded with feigned incredulity, for rhetorical effect: "The unbelievable thing is that this woman accused the victim of theft of having wanted to rape her, as if being raped was a regular habit of hers!" This was also greeted with hilarity, "laughter in the room." The audience was frequently described as "moved" or shocked emotionally by details of the testimonies. For example, audience members' reactions were noted when Pierre Fiquet reported his shock at seeing his wife had put Henriette in the canal: "I was overcome when I saw what she was going to do. (The audience responds with emotion.)" The effect of these journalistic asides was to guide the reader and distance the ordinary men and women in the audience from the exceptional and "monstrous" femme Fiquet.[32]

This double standard was extended in court to some of Fiquet's sexual conquests. During the trial, clearer evidence emerged of the alleged relationships between Fiquet and the doctor Michelot and the Abbé Pihéry. This evidence was used to indict Fiquet, but no comments were made on the reputations of the men involved. Was the assumption that these men, too, were victims of Fiquet's seductions and manipulations? There was also a clear class standard being applied here, which has previously been noted by Harris: "The servant maid and the bourgeois lady received very different responses in court, as did the male working-class laborer and the refined Parisian aesthete."[33] The gentleman's word was considered infallible.

First among the doctors to testify about Fiquet's past actions, illnesses, and simulations was Michelot, who had treated Fiquet at home with morphine injections in 1880. One of the Fiquet family's neighbors, the widow Barbey, was asked under oath whether men or children often went into the family home. She testified that a young doctor (*interne*) used to go "quite frequently" to Fiquet's home and would stay there "for hours on end."[34] This was confirmed in Marie Cagnard's deposition, another neighbor who reported, "She [Fiquet] was called on frequently by doctors and creditors: but for the latter she was never home."[35] When Michelot took the stand, he was only briefly questioned about the femme Fiquet's character and not at all about the nature of his relationship with the woman he was testifying against, the ethics of his own behavior, or his own possible biases due to the liaison. This was a trial in which rumor and hearsay were given the status of objective truth and in which Marie-Françoise Fiquet was judged for her moral reputation as much as for the specific crime she was alleged to have committed.[36]

Second, the trial reports corroborated Fiquet's likely affair with the priest l'Abbé Pihéry, which had occurred in 1879–80. During this time, as we have seen, Fiquet was pregnant and lost a baby. The most damning piece of evidence here was the testimony of the Fiquets' niece, sixteen-year-old Marie Fenet, who had been asked to dispose of what appeared to be the body of a baby, placed in a cotton sack and thrown in the river. Metman, knowing the substance of the affair, "requested that this deposition not be heard, because it is particularly painful for the *femme* Fiquet, and he calls on the humanity of Monsieur le president."[37] This recording of Metman's request was the only time it was suggested, by the femme Fiquet or others, that she had been upset by recalling the events surrounding the death of her baby, and therefore that she had indeed remembered it as a traumatic event.

Contradicting the account the Abbé Pihéry had given in his pretrial statement, in which he claimed to have visited the femme Fiquet only once or twice, Fenet stated that the priest "came often to visit the accused woman." The report continued, "The witness [the niece Marie Fenet] was under instruction, as soon as she saw him arrive, to alert the *femme* Fiquet, who would immediately get undressed and climb into bed, and Father Pierri [*sic*] would enter and the Fenet girl would leave."[38] Fenet, under oath, then told the court what Fiquet had asked her to do. As for Pihéry, he invoked the Seal of the Confessional and was not required to testify. His immunity was therefore complete, although we do not know if the exposure of his behavior in the trial negatively affected his reputation.

The third man who was a significant actor in the story, but who was treated leniently, was Pierre Fiquet. His own depositions stated that he walked to the canal with his wife, although he denied carrying the child or placing her in the water. Key testimonies from neighbors, such as the femme Lefebvre, also depicted him as a good man dominated by a clever, evil woman: "She [Lefebvre] depicts the accused as a negligent woman, who took very little care of her home and none at all of her husband. He got up early in the morning, did the housework, prepared breakfast and went to work, while she stayed at home and didn't lift a finger."[39] Lefebvre saw the femme Fiquet as the clear perpetrator: "I have nothing bad to say about him, I think he was more of a victim."[40]

Pierre Fiquet was consistently presented as a "docile instrument" deployed to serve a criminal mastermind, his wife. His defense lawyer, Cunisset, in his summing up described Pierre Fiquet as irremediably "under the influence of this woman who viewed him merely as a slave."[41] Pierre Fiquet's stupidity, docility, passivity, and essential harmlessness were emphasized throughout proceedings. Where he was rendered weak and submissive, his wife was depicted as assertive and virile. Yet, had the roles been reversed, it is difficult to imagine that a female accomplice would have been treated so leniently.

When Mademoiselle Bautut took the stand to testify about Fiquet's fraudulent attempts to practice midwifery, she offered further insights into the accused woman's predatory behavior. Fiquet first groomed Bautut by approaching her at the town's charitable medical services for the poor; she told the young woman that she could tell just from looking at her face that she was pregnant. Fiquet then allegedly pressured the young woman into purchasing a belt for fifteen francs and, as the report stated, "during one of her last visits, the *femme* Fiquet even practiced maneuvers which could compromise the girl's pregnancy."[42] It is difficult to ascertain what the true nature of this transaction was. Perhaps the Bautut girl had, in fact, sought Fiquet's assistance to procure an abortion. In this instance, she would perhaps not admit this motivation in court. The Fiquet trial was typical, therefore, in how it showed ordinary people being called to give an account of their lives, everyday interactions with others, and the conflicts and troubles that arose as a result. These testimonies were necessary because the lives of women inhabiting the different strata of society were so different, and their experiences needed to be spelled out to the audience.[43]

The président commented on Fiquet's mental clarity and keen intellect, evoking again her criminal artistry, in response to Fiquet's fierce denial of her neighbor Marie Cagnard's earlier testimony. Fiquet remarked that she had a terrible reputation anyway and so had no hope of a fair trial. In response, "M. le président remarked to the *femme* Fiquet that she replies with great lucidity, and even with wit."[44] However, in response to Mademoiselle Bautut's testimony, the président challenged Fiquet about "the gravity of her behavior in presenting herself as a midwife." Although Fiquet did reply, her voice was again erased from the trial report in the press—in some contrast to the medical reports, in which, as we saw in chapter 4, her voice enjoys such prominence: "The accused woman gives quite long explanations that it is pointless to relate."[45] It seemed to be the element of deliberate deception involved in the interaction between the femme Fiquet, a trusted older woman, and the vulnerable Mademoiselle Bautut that the président found so abhorrent.

Gide, in *Souvenirs de la Cour d'assises* (1913), noted that the court président tended to frame questions in a manner likely to be unintelligible to the (typically) undereducated accused person and witnesses. In this case, that Fiquet not only understood but was also capable of engaging in repartee with legal men was surprising to the officials in the courtroom. This explains why her accusers and reporters resorted to accusations of stereotypically feminine prolixity rather than stupidity; it also coheres with the image of Fiquet as a terrifying criminal genius.[46] It was common for defendants' testimonies to be preserved verbatim in the *Gazette des Tribunaux* account of the more prominent trials.[47] As a minor, if briefly sensational, regional affair, the Fiquet case was not recorded in the *Gazette*. This is unfortunate for our purposes because we must instead rely on the summaries, paraphrases, and brief citations included in the local press reports.

As the *Catholique* reported, "The public, whose curiosity had been aroused by the language of certain newspapers," had "flocked to the hearing." On the last day of the trial, a loud mob attempted to invade the courtroom, high with excitement and curiosity, eager to hear the gruesome details of the crime on the final day of testimonies. Inside the courtroom, it reported, "Monsieur le Président often had to quell lively protests." Some press reports even stated that soldiers had to hold the crowd at the door after the public gallery had to be emptied.[48] The trial went on, although the président struggled to maintain order. This mob rage was clearly directed at Marie-Françoise Fiquet, singled out for public shaming.

The reports in the *Démocratie Bourguignonne*, having underlined the incoherence of the femme Fiquet's responses (directly contradicting the président's assessment of her unusual intelligence), concluded by emphasizing the brilliance of both Mairet's and Metman's summing up speeches. For the prosecution, Mairet's lasted almost two hours and was "pronounced with a

VIII. L'*affaire* FIQUET. — Les débats se sont pro-
longés depuis le lundi 5 mars au matin jusqu'au
mercredi 7 à six heures du soir. Le public, dont la
curiosité avait été surexcitée par le langage de cer-
tains journaux, se portait en foule aux audiences ;
le dernier jour les militaires ont eu à repousser pres-
que une tentative d'invasion. Dans l'intérieur, M. le
président a dû comprimer souvent des manifestations
inconsidérées.

Françoise Rémond, née en 1851 dans l'arrondisse-
ment de Gray, a mené jusqu'en 1880 une vie assez
nomade. On la voit à Besançon, à Epinal, à Dijon et
dans différents villages de cette région, vivant comme domestique ou comme ouvrière, mais signalée
de très bonne heure comme adonnée au libertinage,
à la paresse, aux fourberies dangereuses. Dès l'âge
de quinze ans, elle a un enfant naturel. En 1875, à

FIGURE 6.   Reporting of the trial in *Le Catholique*, March 1883. Courtesy of Bibliothèque nationale de France.

firm voice and with the authority of a magistrate charged with defending the
interests of society," greatly impressing the audience.[49] His speech was not
reported in its entirety, and the details of the crime were glossed over; instead,
the stories about Fiquet's immoral lifestyle prior to Henriette's murder were
emphasized. Mairet's opening summary evidenced his approach:

To begin with, who are the accused?

You must certainly have been struck, gentlemen, by the strange
appearance of this creature with a brilliantly intelligent, but hard and
pitiless, gaze, by her energetic, irrepressible, and shrewd personality,
you will have noticed how Marie Rémond, *femme* Fiquet, replied to all
the questions asked, and to all the witness declarations, with such presence of mind and with consummate ease, combining lies and hypocrisy with a shockingly coldblooded attitude. . . . Raised beneath the
African sun, she acquired all its passions: at the age of fifteen, she was
living a shameless life, at seventeen, she was a mother, at twenty-six,
she was convicted of theft and did not hesitate to accuse her victim of

having violated her purity and of having accepted the return of a stolen object in payment for his silence. Soon enough, men fled her presence, driven away by her disgraceful sexual precocity.[50]

Without even mentioning the crime for which Fiquet was standing trial, Mairet drew out selected details, such as her penetrating intelligence, visible from the physiognomic sign of the "look" or "gaze"; her hard, pitiless, energetic, wildly powerful character; and her sangfroid, hypocrisy, and deceptions. There were, of course, other hypocritical, perverted, and dishonest actors in the room who would never be held to account for their actions.

This was also the first time Fiquet's childhood under the "African sun" was invoked, but the exotic connotations of fiery passions were useful to the dramatic portrait and call to mind other racialized portraits of evil murderesses, such as Zola's *Thérèse Raquin* (1868), whose eponymous antiheroine was described as having African blood coursing through her veins. As we saw earlier, Mairet did not believe that promiscuous women could be raped, and therefore Fiquet's "unnatural" actions were cast as motiveless and driven by simple, evil intent. Fiquet's criminal intelligence was aligned with her "disgraceful sexual precocity," through which she was able to remain a step ahead of her victims until her crimes finally caught up with her. All this was pronounced with "the concision and eloquence" for which the lawyer was well known, again contrasting with what the newspapers reported as Fiquet's ill-considered ramblings.

As for Pierre Fiquet, he was simply "a man subjected to the domination, the very tyranny of his wife without uttering a word of protest and who, on 29 June, did not find in his conscience the slightest feeling of resistance or moral outrage against the crime plotted by this woman." He was simply too intellectually deficient to help Henriette and to stand against the evil being perpetrated by his wife.[51] This was sufficient to mark out his guilt, but Mairet did not insist on it strongly; he recommended a guilty verdict but with a largely attenuated punishment. Pierre Fiquet's failure to help the child would have appeared less obviously monstrous than Fiquet's actions due to the gendered interpretation of the crime and the way in which he was presented as the passive victim of her manipulations. This will have indicated anxiety about his diminished masculinity and contributed to the court's relative leniency in his case.

Mairet's speech then considered the "kind" assessment offered by Dr. Blanche of Fiquet's mental condition and concluded by recommending severe punishment with the attenuating circumstances suggested by medical authorities; the femme Fiquet should, Mairet was clear, be spared the ultimate punishment of execution, in recognition of a possible underlying mental disturbance, but should be harshly chastised in reflection of the cruel and callous deed she had committed.

Metman's speech was similarly praised in the press for its lucidity and forensic analysis. However, his arguments for the defense relied equally on establishing the uniqueness of Marie-Françoise Fiquet as a killer. He argued that his client had made no attempt to conceal her actions. She had not set out to kill Henriette; therefore, no evidence of premeditation existed. Crucially, he added, the accused could not be considered "an ordinary criminal." Believing she had been guided by spirits who predestined her for the scaffold, Fiquet was, according to Metman, certainly deranged, even though the medical reports commissioned by the investigation failed to draw that conclusion. Although Metman mentioned her delusions, he said nothing at all about Fiquet's chronic morphine abuse. The skillful defender pointed out the circumstantial and speculative nature of the evidence leveraged in pursuit of Fiquet's conviction, and the problem of a lack of motive. Metman's final speech directly challenged the medical authorities, Blanche and Marandon, who had affirmed after their painstaking examinations that Fiquet was sane and could be considered responsible for her crimes, even with attenuated responsibility.[52]

Metman drew on competing psychiatric theories of hysteria to cast doubt on the experts' assessments, calling Fiquet's urge to acquire children a "mania" that had drawn Henriette into her trap. The recognition that this woman's successful and attempted abductions were rooted in a deep mental disturbance (mania) was the only time in the whole process that any observer pointed to the hypothesis of "simulation"—as Munchausen-type behavior was theorized at that time—as a mental pathology rather than a manifestation of evil. This direct legal challenge to medical authority prefigured later controversial cases, such as the Papin sisters' trial in 1933, in which the domestic maids were convicted of brutally murdering their employer's wife and daughter. The forensic expert in that case, Dr. Truelle, concluded that the sisters were not insane, despite manifest evidence to the contrary, and his verdict was openly criticized by advocates for the defense.[53]

Metman agreed with Blanche's and Marandon's previous assertions that the story about accidental poisoning was plausible and that everything that occurred up until the moment Henriette was taken from the family apartment was "not a crime, but an accident." Fiquet's defender presented the crime as a series of unintended, accidental but connected events that were misunderstood even by their perpetrators. Journalists noted, "Examining next the pathological state of the defendant, the honorable defense lawyer says that she is a hysteric and that she has all the symptoms; he cites various passages drawn from medical works that he has to hand."[54]

Marandon had found in his psychiatric report that these supposedly "hysterical" symptoms were simulations. One wonders what Charcot's assessment would have been, had he taken the brief. There was a conflict, therefore, between medical and legal knowledge, the latter also informed by lay intuition, which was dramatically staged in the trial. The medical reports threatened Fiquet's chance of acquittal, so Metman had nothing to lose in directly challenging their authority by referring to medical texts in his speech. His point was that medical diagnosis, particularly of mental disturbance, was inherently slippery and could not be relied on to convict. Metman's strategy was a common tactic adopted by defense lawyers at this time: rather than a reversal of the likely verdict, he would have been seeking to secure mitigation.[55]

On the final day of proceedings, Marie-Françoise and Pierre Fiquet were judged by a jury of their peers. Pierre Fiquet was acquitted of all charges. Marie-Françoise Rémond, femme Fiquet, was found guilty but with attenuating circumstances, offering some recognition of her pathological but still misunderstood character and the uncertain effects of drug use on her judgment and moral capacity.[56] Although spared execution, Fiquet was condemned to twenty years of hard labor.

French juries were often lenient in cases of abortion and infanticide—increasingly so in the years after 1880, often acquitting women who killed their own babies out of desperation.[57] That juries were slightly less lenient in cases, like the Fiquet affair, where the motivation was so unclear, suggests that there were other factors at play in these instances. In different ways, women like Marie-Françoise Fiquet and Constance Thomas seemed to act out of compulsion and exhibited an appetite for killing that went beyond necessity, desperation, or expediency, and which disturbed the public. Juries could relate to women who sought out abortions or smothered newborns out of misery and despair, but they could not understand killing for money or pleasure, repeatedly, in a calmly ritualized way. Nor could they understand the gratuitous killing of an innocent five-year-old girl, no matter how strange or disturbed the perpetrator.

Despite the sensational nature of the trial, and Fiquet's conviction, the public was left at a point of anticlimax. "The outcome of this case did not satisfy anyone," *La Côte-d'Or* would complain two days later, judging that "it remains mysterious on all points. We know less than ever the motives of the crime, and we do not even know how little Henriette was killed. . . . A well-directed investigation would have brought other results."[58] In some sense, therefore, the crime seems to have remained "unrepresentable," in Kalifa's terms, with the assembled conceptual apparatus available to the decision-makers in this story.

CHAPTER 6

Afterlives

The last word written about the femme Fiquet in the dossier tells us she was condemned to twenty years of hard labor. I expected this to mean transportation to the French penal colonies, in either French Guyana on the northeast coast of South America or New Caledonia in the South Pacific. I began my search with the Archives Nationales d'Outre-Mer in Aix-en-Provence, where the records of those transported overseas into penal servitude are held. The Archives held no record of a woman named Rémond or Fiquet, so it appears unlikely that this had been her fate. It does seem plausible, given her fragile health, that once convicted Fiquet died in prison or hospital in Dijon before serving out her time. In the 1880s, the average life expectancy for a woman who reached adulthood in France was forty-five years, which we might expect to be reduced by extreme poverty, chronic illness, drug dependency, malnutrition, and poor mental health.[1]

Odile Krakovitch is a French historian who, in *Les Femmes bagnardes*, studied the fate of many of the women who were sent to penal colonies. Krakovitch has called the transportation of criminals the great antiprogressive "crime" of the Second Empire (1852–70) and the Third Republic (1870–1940); the United Kingdom, for example, had effectively ended penal transportation in the 1850s. Ten thousand French women prisoners died in the colonies (out of a total of seventy thousand transported, men and women). Of those who returned, only the Communard and socialist-anarchist feminist Louise

Michel left a written testimony. In *Le Livre du bagne* (written between 1872 and 1884), Michel vividly described the harsh conditions of transportation and her comradeship with other female prisoners. Despite the material privations prisoners endured, Michel also evoked the relative freedoms of life in the penal colony (enabling her, for example, to study botany and become politically engaged with the local Indigenous population).[2]

Female political prisoners such as Michel, who were considered subversive and dangerous forces, were forcibly removed to the penal colonies.[3] Other women were given the choice to go or stay: They were allowed to serve their sentence in prison in the Metropole. Men were transported to work, but the motivation for transporting women was to populate the colonies of the future. As a result, the authorities prioritized young (under thirty), robust, healthy women who would travel "willingly" to the colonies.[4] Given this precedent, the femme Fiquet would surely not have been a good candidate for the scheme. Her fate, as with various other aspects of this case, remains a mystery.

The Fiquet affair was one of several medicolegal investigations concerning morphine addiction in fin-de-siècle France that would go on to be cited in the subsequent literature on crime and criminal responsibility. In addition to Marandon's and Blanche's longer reports, the case would be mentioned in several research papers and medical theses published in the decade that followed.[5] It illustrated a consensus among juries and experts that drug addiction did not cause *violent* criminal behavior, although it could trigger behavioral dysregulation among addicts in withdrawal.

Sara Black has argued that the trouble with morphine addiction and its relationship to crime was that it was easily hidden. Many addicts seemed to lead normal lives if they could access their regular doses.[6] In criminal trials, morphine was often viewed as a "normalizing force" that controlled underlying mental disturbances rather than produced them. Therefore, "addiction did not serve as a straightforward legal defense, because doctors recognized the regulatory power of morphine over the addicted body."[7] Logically, therefore, a crime could not be mitigated because a morphine user was experiencing withdrawal symptoms *and* intoxication: It had to be one or the other. In Fiquet's example, the striking elements of her presentation to doctors were the simulation of both physical and psychological symptoms. Marandon was therefore not truly convinced that the femme Fiquet was affected by her drug dependency, whether in withdrawal or not.

Later commentators would repeat Marandon's contradictory assertions about the medicolegal significance of morphine addiction. Henri Guimbail's treatise *Les Morphinomanes* (1892), which contained sections on addiction and cited the Fiquet affair, argued that in the case of morphine abuse, the self was effaced, melted even. Guimbail asserted that this loss of self and free will was so serious that it should be formally recognized as an "excuse" for serious crimes, because "the morphinomaniac loses little by little their moral freedom." Guimbail cited the case of George Henry Lamson, a heavily indebted morphine-addicted doctor who was hanged in London in 1882 for poisoning his brother-in-law to fraudulently obtain his inheritance. Guimbail concluded that morphinomania was "an illness that ruins the body, disturbs the mind, leading its enthusiasts fatally into a brutalized state, often into crime and misdemeanor, and always to martyrdom."[8]

Yet, in the same passage of text, Guimbail referred to Marandon's sound analysis of the Fiquet affair and concluded, with Marandon, that this woman, although avowedly a morphine addict, was fully responsible for her crime. Lamson's crime was motivated by the desire to obtain money to feed a drug habit and was therefore excusable (if regrettable), because it could be understood as an act of desperation linked to the acquisition of morphine. Fiquet's misdeed, however, was rooted in moral perversion, and her morphine addiction was incidental to this. The capacity for murder and a penchant for drug abuse were two sides of a defective character, but the addiction did not cause the moral problem. Guimbail argued that the question of criminal responsibility was complex and that drug use could be viewed as either an aggravating factor or a mitigating factor. Although he conceded that some drugs could occasionally induce moral anesthesia, he ultimately determined that Fiquet was largely responsible for the death of Henriette Barbey.[9]

The same press that had imagined the bereaved family as honest, working-class folk would soon reveal how the Barbey ménage was perfectly dysfunctional in its own way. Henriette's grandmother, the widow Tissot, had written to the examining magistrate, prior to Fiquet's trial, to tell him about her son-in-law's disgraceful behavior and chronic alcoholism.[10] In August 1883, five months after the Fiquet trial was concluded, Athanäse Barbey appeared in court and was convicted of sexually molesting his teenage niece. It would be noted in the press that while in custody he was suffering from delirium tremens because of his alcoholism, corroborating his mother-in-law's accusations. Marandon also observed that the prosecution had for a long time suspected Henriette's parents of involvement in the disappearance of their daughter, calling them "people without morals," despite the press having previously presented them as paragons of working-class virtue.[11]

If there were any lingering doubts about Marie-Françoise Fiquet's obsession with abducting children, two further incidents would come to light after her trial was completed. In a supplementary folder of evidence gathered in early 1883, but too late to be considered during the trial, there are two sets of additional statements that suggested to investigators that Fiquet had previously attempted to abduct young girls. The first episode had occurred in the spring of 1880 when Fiquet (who was then still living in Besançon) traveled some sixty kilometers (thirty-seven miles) to an orphanage in Auxonne and asked to take two girls, Justine and Maria Jobard, then aged eleven and thirteen, into town. Fiquet claimed to be their aunt, but the girls did not recognize her. Despite Fiquet's strong insistence, Sister Clotilde Marie had firmly refused to allow her to take them.[12]

The second incident had occurred on 10 April 1882, two and a half months before Henriette's murder. A little girl, two-year-old Pauline Mugnier, disappeared from the courtyard outside her family's home in the rue Guillaume, northwest of Dijon city center and a short walk from the Fiquet abode, where she had gone to play after lunch. The child was found later in the afternoon abandoned at the city railway station. One witness reported seeing the child there with a small woman, dressed in black, and a man. A letter from the French Railway Board confirmed that Pierre Fiquet was employed at the station at that time, and he had been at work that day.[13] Fiquet had therefore likely rehearsed the abduction of a child before Henriette was taken and had also involved her husband. Perhaps he foiled his wife's abduction attempt on this occasion and persuaded her to leave the child at the railway station.

Marandon de Montyel was a young man when he was charged with examining the femme Fiquet's medical condition, but the issues at stake aligned with interests he would develop throughout his career. Marandon's ideas were progressive on the management of asylums for the insane in France—a subject on which he was somewhat idealistic. He was closely involved in discussions surrounding the establishment of a new asylum at Ville-Évrard, where he was medical director, in 1900. The *British Medical Journal* would report that Marandon "holds that the patients should lead the lives of artisans, agricultural laborers, etc., living under conditions which shall as far as possible realize the idea of a home" in opposition to a majority of the council, who were "in favor of an asylum of the prison or barrack order."[14] By 1886, Marandon was chief physician of Paris public asylums, suggesting that the Fiquet case and his collaboration with Dr. Blanche advanced his career and established his reputation in the capital.[15]

Marandon's idealism and his inclination toward paternalism did at times verge on the authoritarian. For example, he advocated forced treatment for alcoholism, arguing that addicts were incapable of curing themselves or achieving moderation in their drinking habits.[16] Marandon's ideas on asylum reform were developed at length in a piece titled *Le nouvel asile d'aliénés de la seine et les asiles unisexués*. This was a spirited defense of the inclusion of an alcohol treatment unit within the new asylum project for the Seine region, opposing the popular notion that "madness is a cruel illness, deserving of every sympathy, but drunkenness is a shameful vice."[17] Marandon worked toward an understanding of alcoholism as an illness and outlined a special treatment program for alcoholics, advocating early intervention for young patients hospitalized for the first time.

Related to his interest in addiction, self-control, and moral responsibility, Marandon also published on the topic of pathological obsessions. He had, in the Fiquet case, shown an interest in the concept of the idée fixe, although he did not conclude that the femme Fiquet was thus obsessed. Twenty years later, in a 1904 article titled "Obsessions et impulsions," Marandon would make a strong case for the recognition of obsession as a true mental illness affecting criminal responsibility.[18] He argued that obsession was a type of *manie sans délire*, drawing on earlier psychiatric frameworks, and that criminal obsessives were often highly intelligent and appeared perfectly sane to those around them.[19] He observed that even premeditated murders could be the result of an irresistible and obsessive urge, giving the example of pyromania.[20] It is interesting that he did not make this connection in the Fiquet case, between the accused woman's claim to have been driven by impulse and the seemingly calculated nature of her crime.

Marandon's later ideas suggest that he must not, at the time of the Fiquet case, have seen morphine addiction as being as socially and morally disruptive as alcoholism. He did not consider Fiquet to be in the grip of an irresistible, morbid obsession—whether morphine, her strange behavior toward children, her belief in spirit guides, or her fixation with medicine. He framed all these as "simulations" at that time, but perhaps later he would have qualified his views.[21]

He went on to become a regular contributor to the *Archives de l'anthropologie criminelle*, in which he defended both the idea of mental disturbance as a mitigating factor in the assessment of criminal responsibility and the crucial role of alienist doctors in this process.[22] This suggests either that he was genuinely convinced the femme Fiquet was neither insane nor "obsessed" as he understood it or that his views on the possible impact of mental disturbances on criminal actions became more expansive with experience.

Even the most optimistic asylum managers faced the perennial problem of limited resources. According to a 1904 editorial in the *Journal of the American Medical Association*, "Dr. Marandon de Montyel, the head of a large asylum, is quoted as saying that if he and all his colleagues were frank they would confess that it was impossible for them to know their own patients."

This problem would be borne out at Marandon's establishment, the Ville-Évrard asylum, which would become a severely repressive establishment in the decades after his death in 1908—as recorded in the letters of some of its famous residents, such as Antonin Artaud and Camille Claudel, who found themselves forcibly isolated from the outside world.[23]

Studies of analogous cases frame the attention-seeking behavior associated with factitious disorder as a pathology. The Fiquet affair shows that clinicians were, in 1883, a long way from recognizing this as a discrete personality disorder. The reluctance on Marandon's part to understand and explain behaviors that would later come under the label of Munchausen syndrome would be an attitude adopted by subsequent clinicians. Julie Repper has highlighted this avoidance as a problem, because press speculation tends to fill the explanatory void: "Rather than attempting to answer this question in a considered and sensitive manner, it appears that . . . professionals themselves have avoided offering explanations, and newspapers have reflected the horror and fear of the general public by leading 'witch hunts' against suspected nurses who become victimized as a result."[24] The reticence of clinicians is often born of the concern that explaining a phenomenon excuses it. With a crime as singular and emotionally revolting as killing a child, the desire to condemn and eliminate overwhelms the need to explain.

In their summing-up speeches in the trial of the femme Fiquet, Metman and Mairet reached similar conclusions in a roundabout way. Both found the crime to be inexplicable, in terms of motive, and considered Fiquet's behavior to be the exception to "normal" femininity. Both gave explanations based on the perception of perversion and insanity, and both achieved narrative coherence by asserting her absolute lucidity, or her absolute madness, rather than recognizing the ambiguity of the situation and the ordinariness of Fiquet's prior suffering coupled with the extraordinariness of her reactions. But, in an adversarial judicial context, we cannot expect to see the nuances and complexities of the case reflected because they did not serve the purpose of the trial. There were only losers in the Fiquet affair. Like Violette Nozière and the Papin sisters, Marie-Françoise Fiquet can be framed as a perpetrator but also as a victim of her own pathological disorder, whether in medical, class, or feminist terms. Women, and the poor working classes, were never entirely powerless, but they were vulnerable to many forces beyond their control, and they suffered in unique and unseen ways. Yet, we are still left with what Marandon termed the "grave lacuna" in the investigation: Where was the motive?

I have suggested that this motive was unknown consciously to Fiquet but that her words and fragmented explanations have given us important insights into her life, her pain, her trauma, and her suffering that point to the source of the impulse that drove her to destroy. There was nothing exceptional about what Marie-Françoise Fiquet experienced as a poor, working woman who lost, killed, or aborted her babies. The more singular aspect to her case was her response to these events and her apparent compulsion to revisit the site of her trauma. Her experiences seemed to trigger a mechanism that led to destructive behavior patterns, the quelling of her pain through morphine use, and a drive to poison and kill.

The perverse solution she brought to the problem of her losses and suffering was twofold: On the one hand, the pleasant anesthesia of daily morphine use was a selfish indulgence that took her away from her pains; on the other, she sought in her behavior to control uncontrollable aspects of her life for reasons that have been observed in the cases of other women criminals too. For a while, this solution "worked," but in the end the walls of the defensive edifice she had erected collapsed around her. She poisoned and murdered, as did similar women, in a tragic and distorted attempt to put her life back in order. The verdict reached, in the context of the limitations of the criminal justice system in which it was made, was probably fair, and the jury also clearly felt there was coherence between natural justice and the truth of events that day. Yet the enduring tragedy of the case is that the precise reasons for Henriette's death could not be understood either, even by her killer.

Above all, however, the conceptual thread that winds its way through the elements of the Fiquet affair is that of a woman who violated key cultural codes of femininity. Marie-Françoise Fiquet was, in the public imagination, supposed to be a woman who cared for children and others. Instead, she injured, harmed, and killed them. In her behavior, she also dared to enact a gender role reversal. Her violent and predatory behavior was therefore cast as virile, where her docile and emasculated husband was neutralized by her power, symbolically castrated.

The focus on the monstrous nature of Fiquet's crime overshadowed most people's consideration of her psychological trauma, her claims about her struggle with addiction to morphine, and the extent to which this dependency was linked to her physical and mental pain. Was it also the final source of pressure that caused her behavior to reel out of control? Violent crimes were always difficult to justify or explain in the case of morphine addicts because, as we have seen, the drug was thought to be a pacifier. The quiet brutality of the femme Fiquet's crime, and the fact that her victim was a child, made people unwilling to consider possible explanations for her behavior, even as they were searching for a motive that could make a woman act so unnaturally, against the rules of nature. As we have seen, her own account of her actions and the evidence gathered from witnesses reveal a complex picture of psychological disturbance embedded in a compulsion to repeat and a mania for control.

So what really happened on the afternoon of 29 June 1882? Like the investigators at the time, we will never be certain, but we can hypothesize based on the totality of the evidence available, interpreted in the context of the complex class and gender dynamics that were a feature of nineteenth-century criminal investigations. Any theory must be based on Fiquet's own account of her actions, which offered the principal key to meaning and understanding. If her attack on Henriette Barbey was premeditated, it was only to the extent that she described experiencing a repeated urge to acquire children and to interfere with them.

It seems most likely that at midday on 29 June, feeling disappointed by her failure to gain legitimate access to the midwifery profession and despairing at her husband's return from hospital, the femme Fiquet acted on a familiar impulse when she coaxed Henriette away from the school gates and persuaded the girl to go home with her. Given Henriette's timid personality, it is likely that she was carried along by events and that Fiquet took the lead in whatever happened that day. The femme Fiquet's recorded history of attempted poisoning and "administering" of medicines make it most likely that she gave Henriette some of the sugared morphine solution, either to sedate the girl and keep her quiet or simply to respond to her own repeated and inexplicable urge to inflict medical procedures on others. Henriette probably fell asleep, sedated. Fiquet woke her late in the evening and walked her to the canal side, where she pushed the child into the water, holding her little head under the surface with an umbrella until she stopped struggling. Pierre Fiquet had followed her and, realizing the gravity of what his wife had done, fled the next day.

The killing, in the end, does seem particularly gratuitous. Marie-Françoise Fiquet could have abandoned Henriette in the street and gone back home, and perhaps she would have remained undiscovered until the next time. But the events of Fiquet's young adult life seem inexorably to have been leading to this event. An untimely human death is said to be a tragedy because it is inevitable yet sometimes the result of imperfect human nature. Fiquet was morally flawed, but the darkness of her character and her capacity for violence had deep roots. Some of these were entwined with the early, arbitrary losses that she experienced as a woman. Others, however, were plausibly triggered by the stressful conditions in which she lived. For Fiquet's contemporaries, she was an exception to be weeded out and eliminated rather than a typical, suffering woman whose story revealed so much about how poor, working women and children lived and died in late nineteenth-century France.

The human need to stigmatize, exclude, root out, and shun is born of the recognizability and the ordinariness of the perpetrator. We are horrified by the possibility that we, too, hold the capacity for violence and cruelty under certain circumstances. Yet this is arguably the truth. Psychiatrist Robert Jay Lifton, an American Jew who lived through the Second World War and who, at the time of writing, is still alive, spent years patiently interviewing German doctors who had participated in practices of mass extermination. Lifton's extraordinary book, *The Nazi Doctors*, demonstrated that atrocities are produced by circumstance and "need not require emotions as extreme or demonic as would seem appropriate for such a malignant project."[25] In the case of the Nazi project of the 1930s and 1940s, one necessary condition was the rationalization of murder through a conceptual reversal of the ideas of healing and killing. Restoring the nation could only be achieved by putting people to death. This was "healing work" because those deemed unworthy of life—the physically weak, the mad, the racially inferior—were "already dead."[26] At the heart of this attitude is an intense desire for order, an anxiety to control the forces of chaos that move through the world. Similarly, Marie-Françoise Fiquet and certain other women like her were subject to the same kind of reversal; they were transformed from mothers and carers into killers. Surely their actions, too, were motivated by a desire to impose order and control over an unpredictable universe.

Krakovitch has argued that women's crimes followed predictable patterns and that much of the femme Fiquet's behavior was, in criminal terms, unexceptional: "Women's crimes were more defensive than offensive, and were a response to an attempt to survive in a hostile environment. Crimes such as infanticide and murder stemmed more from an inability to cope with life and its difficulties than from a desire for power and wealth, or a desire to rebel."[27] Extensive research into this single case has led me to draw parallels between Marie-Françoise Fiquet and other cases of women with similar background experiences and behavioral profiles who also ran into trouble with the law. I have argued that Marie-Françoise Fiquet exhibited most if not all of the known symptoms of a factitious disorder and that the loss of at least two babies, before birth or during infancy, was probably a significant psychological stressor in her life.

Further research would likely reveal that factitious disorders were both more common than has previously been recognized and clustered among women with similar social profiles. I would expect to find that many historic cases of midwives, abortionists, and baby farmers who ran into legal trouble exhibited elements of this troubled psychological profile. It is also possible that carrying out these activities led some women, with specific vulnerabilities, to *develop* factitious disorders as a response to the stress of dealing with the vicissitudes of pregnancy, childbirth, and infant care. They would often have been women who had their own babies young, in their teens and early twenties, and who thus gained experience of caring for infants early in life. Women with factitious disorders would have been indistinguishable from other people working as midwives and nurses, simply because the lines were so impossibly blurred and because their actions would rarely have come under legal scrutiny. It is easy for helping and nurturing to tip into suffocating and controlling behavior, meaning that factitious disorder must necessarily be a spectrum.

It was in this murky, gray area between struggling and coping, neglecting and caring, that women like the femme Fiquet operated, and it was precisely because the truth was so hard to pin down that their actions, when discovered, elicited strong public responses of disgust and horror—as did poisoning. These women will always walk among us, and tragedies are impossible to avert altogether. Yet the case of Marie-Françoise Fiquet shows us that the unique stresses of young, working women's lives in provincial France, during a time of dynamic social change, produced a specific type of woman and a specific type of violence.

NOTES

Introduction

1. According to reports in *La Démocratie Bourguignonne*, 1 July 1882.

2. Henri Gallimard statement, 6 July 1882. All statements cited are located in the Archives Départementales de la Côte-d'Or (ADCO), 2 U 1495.

3. One witness who was at the canal side, Bonaventure, described the evening as "quite dark" in his statement given on 31 July 1882.

4. Francine Barreau statement, 30 June 1882.

5. For an excellent and comprehensive history, see Jean-Noël Luc, *L'invention du jeune enfant au XIXe siècle: De la salle d'asile à l'école maternelle* (Belin, 1997).

6. Louise Coquereaux statement, 30 June 1882.

7. Frédéric Huppert statement, 30 June 1882.

8. The information that follows on the political positions of the newspapers cited is from Émile Mermet's comprehensive directory, the *Annuaire de la presse française* (Chez l'auteur, 1883).

9. "Un crime mystérieux à Dijon," *La Démocratie Bourguignonne*, 1 July 1882.

10. "Un crime mystérieux à Dijon," *Le Bien Public*, 1 July 1882. When I was researching the case, the left-wing popular daily, the *Petit Bourguignon*, was not available for consultation at the Bibliothèque nationale de France due to its poor condition.

11. A concept analyzed by Louis Chevalier in *Classes laborieuses et classes dangereuses à Paris pendant la première moitié du XIXe siècle* (Plon, 1958).

12. My emphasis.

13. "Le crime de Dijon," *Le Catholique*, 1 and 8 July 1882.

14. See chap. 2 on the investigation.

15. "Le crime de Dijon," *La Démocratie Bourguignonne*, 1–4 July 1882.

16. "Le crime de Dijon," *La Démocratie Bourguignonne*, 7 July 1882.

17. "Le crime de Dijon," *Le Catholique*, 1 July 1882.

18. "Un crime mystérieux à Dijon," *Le Progrès*, 1 July 1882. These details even appeared in the Parisian press: Those reporting the apparent bruising to the child's head from 3 to 5 July 1882 (the week following the murder) included *Gil Blas*, *Le Gaulois*, *Le Petit Parisien*, and *Le Temps*.

19. Dr. Deroye, autopsy report, 6 July 1882.

20. Michel Foucault, ed., *Moi, Pierre Rivière, ayant égorgé ma mère, ma sœur et mon frère . . .: Un cas de parricide au XIXe siècle* (Gallimard/Julliard, 1973), 269.

21. On the question of criminal responsibility and mental disturbance, also see Ruth Harris, *Murders and Madness: Medicine, Law, and Society in the Fin de Siècle* (Clarendon, 1989).

22. Thomas Dormandy, *Opium: Reality's Dark Dream* (Yale University Press, 2012), 120; Howard Padwa, *Social Poison: The Culture and Politics of Opiate Control in Britain and France, 1821–1926* (Johns Hopkins University Press, 2012), 40–41.

23. Jean-Jacques Yvorel, "La loi du 12 juillet 1916," *Les cahiers dynamiques* 56, no. 3 (2012): 128–33. On the international conventions designed to control access to drugs, see Virginia Berridge, *Opium and the People: Opiate Use and Policy in Nineteenth and Early Twentieth Century England* (Free Association, 1999), 239–42.

24. Jean-Jacques Yvorel, *Les poisons de l'esprit: Drogues et drogués au XIX* Siècle* (Quai Voltaire, 1992), 237–41; Emmanuelle Retaillaud-Bajac, *Les paradis perdus: Drogues et usagers de drogues dans la France de l'entre-deux-guerres* (Presses Universitaires de Rennes, 2009), 10–11.

25. Terry M. Parssinen and Karren Kerner, "Development of the Disease Model of Drug Addiction in Britain, 1870–1926," *Medical History* 24, no. 3 (1980): 275–96.

26. On the profile of nineteenth-century addicts in America, see chap. 2 of David. T. Courtwright, *Dark Paradise: A History of Opiate Addiction in America* (Harvard University Press, 2001).

27. Dr. Marandon de Montyel, "De la morphinomanie dans ses rapports avec la médecine légale," *L'Encéphale* 3, no. 1 (1881): 669. The asylum was an old Carthusian monastery and is sometimes called "la Chartreuse" (in reference to the building) and sometimes called "l'asile des Chartreux," in reference to the former residents.

28. Marandon, "De la morphinomanie," 702.

29. Anna Motz, *A Love That Kills: Stories of Forensic Psychology and Female Violence* (Weidenfeld & Nicolson, 2023), 4.

1. Approaches

1. Foucault, *Moi, Pierre Rivière*, 9–10.

2. For an excellent discussion of role and purpose of the *fait divers*, see Sarah C. Maza, *Violette Nozière: A Story of Murder in 1930s Paris* (University of California Press, 2011), 144–45.

3. See chapter 4 of Harris, *Murders and Madness*, on the tensions between medical and legal knowledge.

4. Philippe Artières, "Crimes écrits: La collection d'autobiographies de criminels du Professeur A. Lacassagne," *Genèses: Sciences Sociales et Histoire* (1995): 48–67.

5. Rachel G. Fuchs, *Poor and Pregnant in Paris: Strategies for Survival in the Nineteenth Century* (Rutgers University Press, 1992), 5.

6. Natalie Zemon Davis, *The Return of Martin Guerre* (Harvard University Press, 2001).

7. Sarah Maza writes, "Microhistory has three defining traits: it concerns a non-famous person or group of people; it centers on a crisis; and the author uses the story to make a point about some broader historical question such as . . . the relation between elite and popular culture." *Thinking About History* (University of Chicago Press, 2017), 178–85.

8. Emmanuel Le Roy Ladurie, *Montaillou, village Occitan de 1294 à 1324* (Gallimard, 1975); Carlo Ginzburg, *The Cheese and the Worms: The Cosmos of a Sixteenth-*

Century Miller, trans. John A. Tedeschi and Anne Tedeschi (Penguin, 1992); Carlo Ginzburg, "Checking the Evidence: The Judge and the Historian," *Critical Inquiry* 18, no. 1 (1991): 79–92.

9. Carlo Ginzburg and Carlo Poni, "La micro-histoire," *Le Débat* 17, no. 10 (1981): 133–36.

10. Edward Berenson, *The Trial of Madame Caillaux* (University of California Press, 1992), 7–8.

11. Robert Finlay, "The Refashioning of Martin Guerre," *American Historical Review* 93, no. 3 (June 1988): 553–71; John H. Arnold, "The Historian as Inquisitor: The Ethics of Interrogating Subaltern Voices," *Rethinking History* 2, no. 3 (1998): 379–86; Dominic LaCapra, *History and Criticism* (Cornell University Press, 1985).

12. Motz, *Love That Kills*.

13. Lisa Downing, *The Subject of Murder: Gender, Exceptionality, and the Modern Killer* (University of Chicago Press, 2013).

14. Anna Norris, *L'écriture du défi: Textes carcéraux féminins du XIXᵉ et du XXᵉ siècles: Entre l'aiguille et la plume* (Summa, 2003); Mary S. Hartman, *Victorian Murderesses: A True History of Thirteen Respectable French and English Women Accused of Unspeakable Crimes* (Robson, 1977).

15. Michelle Perrot, "Ouverture," in *Femmes et justice pénale: XIXᵉ–XXᵉ siècles*, ed. Christine Bard et al. (Presses universitaires de Rennes, 2002), 9–21; Ann-Louise Shapiro, *Breaking the Codes: Female Criminality in Fin-de-Siècle Paris* (Stanford University Press, 1996), 4.

16. Perrot, "Ouverture," 9–21.

17. Shapiro, *Breaking the Codes*, 4, 14.

18. Elissa D. Gelfand, *Imagination in Confinement: Women's Writings from French Prison* (Cornell University Press, 1983), 42.

19. Raymond de Ryckère, *La femme en prison et devant la mort: Étude de criminologie* (A. Storck, 1898). Cesare Lombroso and Guglielmo Ferrero, *La donna delinquente, la prostitua e la donna normale* (Editori L. Roux, 1893), translated into English (without the section on "normal" woman) as Lombroso and Ferrero, *The Female Offender* (Appleton, 1900); Camille Granier, *La femme criminelle* (O. Doin, 1906).

20. Joëlle Guillais, *Crimes of Passion: Dramas of Private Life in Nineteenth-Century France* (Polity, 1990), 182–86.

21. Shapiro, *Breaking the Codes*, 20.

22. André Gide, *Ne jugez pas* (Gallimard, 1957); Foucault, *Moi, Pierre Rivière*.

23. A point most poignantly made in Truman Capote, *In Cold Blood: A True Account of a Multiple Murder and Its Consequences* (Random House, 1965). Capote analyzed the brutal 1959 murder of four members of the Herbert Clutter family in Kansas.

24. Harris, *Murders and Madness*, 21; Hartman (*Victorian Murderesses*) and Maza (*Violette Nozière*) also make this point. See also Eliza Earle Ferguson, *Gender and Justice: Violence, Intimacy, and Community in Fin-de-Siècle Paris* (Johns Hopkins University Press, 2010). Ferguson (2) has found that acquittal rates for women tried in the assizes courts at the turn of the century were as high as 64 percent and that this was due to leniency in cases of intimate violence.

25. Rachel Edwards and Keith Reader, *The Papin Sisters* (Oxford University Press, 2001); Maza, *Violette Nozière*.

26. Ferguson, *Gender and Justice*, 13–14.

27. Berenson, *Trial of Madame Caillaux*, 92.

28. Jan Goldstein, *Hysteria Complicated by Ecstasy: The Case of Nanette Leroux* (Princeton University Press, 2010).

29. Critics have not historically agreed on where the line should be drawn between prostitutes and courtesans, if at all. Charles Bernheimer has argued that a courtesan is "a prostitute who associates with men of wealth and prestige." See *Figures of Ill Repute: Representing Prostitution in Nineteenth-Century France* (Duke University Press, 1997), 6–7. Mireille Dottin-Orsini makes a stronger distinction, drawing on Corbin's analysis, and argues there was a gulf of experience between the powerful courtesan and the poor, exploited street prostitute. See Mireille Dottin-Orsini and Daniel Grojnowski, *L'imaginaire de la prostitution: De la Bohème à la Belle Époque* (Paris, 2017), 16–17. Interestingly, Corbin conceptualizes prostitution as an entire economy containing multitudes of experience. See Alain Corbin, *Les filles de noce: Misère sexuelle et prostitution* (Flammarion, 1982).

30. Sarah Horowitz, "Scandalous Friendships: The Dangers of Intimacy in the Steinheil Affair of 1908–1909," *Romanic Review* 110, nos. 1–4 (2019): 252.

31. Elizabeth Comack and Salena Brickey, "Constituting the Violence of Criminalized Women," *Canadian Journal of Criminology and Criminal Justice* 49, no. 1 (January 2007): 1–2.

32. *Kaplan & Sadock's Comprehensive Textbook of Psychiatry*, ed. Benjamin J. Sadock et al. (Wolters Kluwer, 2017). See section 19 on Factitious Disorder.

33. Michel Botbol and Adeline Gourbil, "The Place of Psychoanalysis in French Psychiatry," *BJPsych International* 15, no. 1 (2018): 3–5.

34. American Psychiatric Association, *Diagnostic and Statistical Manual of Mental Disorders*, 5th ed., 2013, 300.19 (F68.10). See also "Factitious Disorder" in Harrison et al., *Shorter Oxford Textbook of Psychiatry*, 7th ed. (Oxford University Press, 2018).

35. Roy Meadow, "Munchausen Syndrome by Proxy: The Hinterland of Child Abuse," *Lancet* 310, no. 8033 (1977): 343–45.

36. Julie Repper, "Munchausen Syndrome by Proxy in Health Care Workers," *Journal of Advanced Nursing* 21, no. 2 (1995): 299–304. John Stirling et al., "Beyond Munchausen Syndrome by Proxy: Identification and Treatment of Child Abuse in a Medical Setting," *Pediatrics* 119, no. 5 (2007): 1026–30.

37. *Kaplan & Sadock's Comprehensive Textbook of Psychiatry*, section 19.

38. The original descriptions of Munchausen syndrome and Munchausen by proxy (by Asher and Meadow) do not suggest that the disorder is brought on by trauma; they imply that it is a type of personality disorder.

39. Hector Gavin, *On Feigned and Factitious Diseases* (J. Churchill, 1843), 3.

40. See, for example, Wolfgang Derblich, *Des maladies simulées dans l'armée et des moyens de les reconnaître*, trans. Adrien Schmit (Asselin, 1883); Paul Chavigny, *Diagnostique des maladies simulées dans les accidents du travail et devant les Conseils de révision et de réforme de l'armée et de la marine* (Baillère, 1906); F. E. Fodéré, *Essai médico-légal sur les diverses espèces de folie vraie, simulée et raisonnée* (L. F. Le Roux, 1832); J. Huguet, *Recherches sur les maladies simulées et mutilations volontaires* (H. Charles-Lavauzelle, 1900); M. Le Professeur Charcot, *Clinique des maladies du système nerveux (1889–90)* (Progrès médical, 1890); Karl A. Menninger, "Psychology of a Certain Type of Malingering," *Archives of Neurology and Psychiatry* 33 (1935): 507–15.

41. Edmond Boisseau, *Des maladies simulées et des moyens de les reconnaitre* (Baillière, 1870).

42. Richard Kanaan and Simon C. Wessely, "The Origins of Factitious Disorder," *History of the Human Sciences* 23, no. 2 (2010): 69–73.

43. Kanaan and Wessely, "Origins of Factitious Disorder," 71; on the medicalization of the life cycle and its unintended consequences, see also Ivan Illich, *Limits to Medicine: Medical Nemesis* (Boyars, 1976).

44. On nostalgia, see Thomas Dodman, *What Nostalgia Was: War, Empire, and the Time of a Deadly Emotion* (University of Chicago Press, 2018).

45. Chris Millard, "Concepts, Diagnosis and the History of Medicine: Historicising Ian Hacking and Munchausen Syndrome," *Social History of Medicine* 30, no. 3 (2017): 567–89.

46. Ian Hacking, *Historical Ontology* (Harvard University Press, 2004), 100–101. The citations here are from the section on "Making Up People."

47. Ian Hacking, *Mad Travelers: Reflections on the Reality of Transient Mental Illnesses* (Harvard University Press, 2002), 7, 18.

48. Hacking, *Historical Ontology*, 111.

49. Kanaan and Wessely, "Origins of Factitious Disorder," 72–73. Although Charcot always believed he was looking for a physiological illness in hysteria, the absence of evidence for this caused these later theorists (Freud, Janet, Menninger) to abandon the idea and treat it as a psychological condition, not a neurological disease.

50. Roland Coutanceau and Joanna Smith, *Troubles de la personnalité: Ni psychotiques, ni névrotiques, ni pervers, ni normaux . . .* (Dunod, 2013).

51. Charcot, *Clinique des maladies du système nerveux*; Josef Breuer and Sigmund Freud, "Studies on Hysteria," in *The Standard Edition of the Complete Psychological Works of Sigmund Freud (Vol. II, 1893–1895)*, ed. and trans. J. Strachey et al. (Hogarth, 1953–1974).

52. Kanaan and Wessely, "Origins of Factitious Disorder," 74.

53. Caroline Eliacheff, "Le syndrome de Münchausen par procuration psychique," *Figures de la psychanalyse* 2, no. 12 (2005): 151–53.

54. For a detailed exploration of these developments, see Jonathyne Briggs, "From Collaboration to Resistance: The Family Dynamic in Autism Literature in Contemporary France," *Contemporary European History* 32, no. 2 (2023): 254–69.

55. For example, Motz makes this case in *A Love That Kills*.

56. Ian Hacking, "Making Up People," *London Review of Books* 28, no. 16 (2006).

57. Sigmund Freud, "Beyond the Pleasure Principle, Group Psychology and Other Works," in *The Standard Edition of the Complete Psychological Works of Sigmund Freud (Vol. XVIII, 1920–22)*, ed. and trans. J. Strachey (Hogarth, 1953–1974).

58. For an exploration of these themes, see Jean-Michel Rabaté, "From the History of Perversion to the Trauma of History," in *The Cambridge Introduction to Literature and Psychoanalysis* (Cambridge University Press, 2014): 174–98.

59. Cathy Caruth, *Unclaimed Experience: Trauma, Narrative, and History* (Johns Hopkins University Press, 2007): 1–6.

60. Ruth Leys, *Trauma: A Genealogy* (University of Chicago Press, 2000), 10.

61. Leys, *Trauma*, 8–10.

62. *Kaplan & Sadock's Comprehensive Textbook of Psychiatry*, section 19.

63. *Kaplan & Sadock's Comprehensive Textbook of Psychiatry*, section 19.

64. I draw the concept of the "control paradox" from the study of anorexia nervosa in Marilyn Lawrence, "Anorexia Nervosa: The Control Paradox," *Women's Studies International Quarterly* 2 (1979): 93–101.

65. Dominique Kalifa, "Les femmes, le crime et l'enquête en France à la fin du XIXᵉ siècle," in *Femmes et Justice Pénale*, ed. Christine Bard et al. (Presses universitaires de Rennes, 2002), 283–92.

66. M. Brady Brower, *Unruly Spirits: The Science of Psychic Phenomena in Modern France* (University of Illinois Press, 2010). This book argues that scientific knowledge was a central pillar of French Third Republic ideology.

67. Arlette Farge, *The Allure of the Archives*, trans. Thomas Scott-Railton (Yale University Press, 2013), 26.

68. Ginzburg, "Checking the Evidence," 91.

69. Farge, *Allure of the Archives*, 93.

2. The Investigation

1. According to the 1872 census (officially the 1871 census, which was delayed by one year due to the Franco-Prussian War). The census data are drawn from the French office of national statistics (INSEE) and recorded as part of a project mapping the evolution of the French population across villages and towns at the École des hautes études en sciences sociales (EHESS): "Des villages de Cassini aux communes d'aujourd'hui: Territoires et Population, deux siècles d'évolution." http://cassini .ehess.fr/fr/html/fiche.php?select_resultat=11845#top.

2. https://www.insee.fr/fr/statistiques/2011101?geo=COM-21231 and https://www.insee.fr/fr/statistiques/4277602?sommaire=4318291.

3. Henri Chabeuf, *Dijon à travers les âges* (Damidot frères, 1897).

4. Chabeuf, *Dijon à travers les âges*, 197–99.

5. Michel Porret, *Le sang des lilas: Une mère mélancolique égorge ses quatre enfants en mai 1885 à Genève* (Georg éditeur, 2019), 26.

6. "Le crime de Dijon," *La Démocratie Bourguignonne*, 2 July 1882.

7. "Assises de la Côte-d'Or," *Le Progrès de la Côte-d'Or*, 2 December 1882.

8. Émile Zola was also liberal in his use of feline metaphors to describe oversexed women, notably in his novel *Thérèse Raquin* (1867).

9. As Bernheimer (*Figures of Ill Repute*, 248) asserts, phallic woman is "the woman become man by the force of her sexual desire."

10. Mireille Dottin-Orsini, *Cette femme qu'ils disent fatale: Textes et images de la misogynie fin-de-siècle* (Bernard Grasset, 1993), 17. Emphasis mine. On the overuse of descriptors such as "serpentine" and "sinuous" to emphasize the bestiality of women, see also Bram Dijkstra, *Idols of Perversity: Fantasies of Feminine Evil in Fin-de-Siècle Culture* (Oxford University Press, 1986), 305.

11. Dottin-Orsini, *Cette femme*, 192 (on the Concile de Mâcon and discussion of women's souls), 275–77. This suggestion reflects the cataloguing of the images of the femme fatale and vampires in Mario Praz, *The Romantic Agony*, 2nd ed. (Oxford University Press, 1970).

12. Dijkstra, *Idols of Perversity*, 331.

13. ADCO, 2 U 1495. "Note" signed "Les agents" [signature illegible]. 30 June 1882.

14. Henri Gallimard statement, 6 July 1882.

15. "Affaire Fiquet," *La Côte-d'Or*, 3 July 1882. The same image of girls dressed in white was reported in *Le Bien Public*.

16. "Assises de la Côte-d'Or," *La Démocratie Bourguignonne*, 2 July 1882.

17. Michelle Perrot, "L'affaire Troppmann (1869)," *L'Histoire* 1981, no. 30 (1981): 28–37, 31.

18. "Assises de la Côte-d'Or," *La Démocratie Bourguignonne*, 2 July 1882.

19. Downing, *Subject of Murder*, 23.

20. "Assises de la Côte-d'Or," *Le Catholique*, 8 July 1882.

21. "Affaire Fiquet," *La Côte-d'Or*, 4 July 1882.

22. The twentieth-century British cases of Myra Hindley, one of the so-called Moors Murderers, and Maxine Carr, the girlfriend of child murderer Ian Huntley, are illustrative of this trend. Neither Hindley nor Carr killed anyone but both were treated as monstrous scapegoats for the actions of their respective male partners in the British tabloid press. For an excellent in-depth discussion of these cases, see chap. 4 of Downing, *Subject of Murder*, on "infanticidal femininity."

23. Philippe Lejeune, "Crime et testament: Les autobiographies de criminels au XIXᵉ Siècle," *Récits de vie & institutions*, nos. 8–9 (1986): 73–98.

24. Athanäse Barbey statement, 30 June 1882.

25. ADCO 2 U 1333, Cours d'appel et d'assisses, mag. M tr. 123, ta. 2, case number 8, 7 March 1883.

26. For a detailed breakdown of "felonies against persons" in the *code penal*, see Benjamin F. Martin, *Crime and Criminal Justice Under the Third Republic: The Shame of Marianne* (Louisiana State University Press, 1990).

27. Henri Gallimard statement, 6 July 1882.

28. Henri Gallimard statement, 20 July 1882.

29. Edmé Michel statement, 11 July 1882.

30. Shapiro, *Breaking the Codes*, 50–51.

31. Shapiro, *Breaking the Codes*, 86.

32. La Femme Fiquet, 1st, 2nd, and 3rd interrogations, and Louise Fiquet statement, 1 July 1882.

33. La Femme Fiquet, 1st interrogation.

34. La Femme Fiquet, 2nd interrogation.

35. La Femme Fiquet, 3rd interrogation.

36. Athanäse Barbey statement, 10 October 1882. Fiquet's statements taken in the first few days following the murder, from 1 to 3 July, deny all involvement and knowledge of the crime.

37. La Femme Fiquet, 5th and 6th interrogations.

38. La Femme Fiquet, 7th interrogation.

39. La Femme Fiquet, 8th interrogation.

40. La Femme Fiquet, 9th interrogation.

41. La Femme Fiquet, 10th interrogation.

42. La Femme Fiquet, 15th interrogation.

43. Pierre Fiquet, 1st interrogation, 1 July 1882.

44. Pierre Fiquet, 2nd interrogation, 2 July 1882.

45. Pierre Fiquet, 2nd interrogation, 2 July 1882.

46. Pierre Fiquet, 2nd interrogation, 2 July 1882. Pierre Fiquet mentioned the name of the village where his parents lived, but it is illegible in the script.

47. See Fuchs, *Poor and Pregnant in Paris*, chaps. 1–2; on the Civil Code, see 37.

48. This is repeated in Marie Fenet's statement, taken on 15 July in Dole.

49. On the evolution of these two views of women, see Gayle K. Brunelle and Annette Finley-Croswhite, *Murder in the Métro: Lætitia Toureaux and the Cagoule in 1930s France* (Louisiana State University Press, 2010), 64–65.

50. Pierre Fiquet, 4th interrogation, 5 July 1882.

51. See Pierre Fiquet, 8th and 9th interrogations, both 24 July 1882.

52. Pierre Fiquet, 10th interrogation, 2 August 1882.

53. See, for example, Asher, "Munchausen's Syndrome," and *Kaplan & Sadock's Comprehensive Textbook of Psychiatry*.

54. Femme Fiquet, letter to Loiseau, 24 July 1882.

55. Deroye, "Rapport" (autopsy report), 6 July 1882; Héberd and Deroye, "Rapport d'experts," (chemical analysis report), 19 July 1882.

56. Louise Fiquet statement (given in Besançon, where she was living with her grandmother), 20 October 1882; Femme Fiquet 8th interrogation, 11 July 1882; Marie Fenet statement (given in Dole, Jura), 15 July 1882.

57. See Sara E. Black, "Morphine on Trial: Legal Medicine and Criminal Responsibility in the Fin de Siècle," *French Historical Studies* 42, no. 4 (2019): 623–53, 633. Black cites contemporary case studies of significant morphine addiction at far lower doses than this.

58. Vincent Schettine statement, 27 July 1882.

59. Black, "Morphine on Trial," 625.

60. Dr. Régnier, *L'intoxication chronique par la morphine et ses diverses formes* (Progrès Medical, 1890), cited in a drug "memoir" by the pseudonymous Comte d'Almond, *Six années de morphinomanie* (Éditions du livre moderne, 1910). Some examples of fictional representations that show characters consuming up to two grams daily include Victorien du Saussay, *La Morphine: Roman passionel* (A. Méricant, 1906); René Schwaeblé, *Les Voluptés de la morphine* (Bibliothèque de l'inconnu, 1908).

61. "La rue Musette et l'église Notre-Dame à Dijon," *Le Bien Public*, 27 August 2017. https://www.bienpublic.com/edition-dijon-ville/2017/08/27/la-rue-musette -et-l-eglise-notre-dame-a-dijon.

62. Gras, *Histoire de Dijon*, 416, and illustration XXIII, "Affiches commerciales des environs 1900," 304–5.

63. Alfred Loiseau, Procès-verbal (report), 1 July 1882.

64. Héberd report, 20 July 1882.

65. Louise Fiquet statement, 1 July 1882.

66. Louise Fiquet statement (given in Besançon, where she was living with her grandmother), 20 October 1882.

67. Letter from Louise Fiquet to her mother, 31 December [1882].

68. Letter from Louise Fiquet to her mother, 31 December [1882]; letter from Louise Fiquet to the examining magistrate, 16 November 1882.

69. Farge, *Allure of the Archives*, 7.

70. Sophie Vaillant statement, 7 October 1882.

71. Femme Tissot statement, 10 October 1882.

72. Femme Barbey statement, 10 October 1882.

73. Athanäse Barbey statement, 10 October 1882.

74. Femme Fiquet, 12th interrogation.

3. The Character Assessment

1. James M. Donovan, *Juries and the Transformation of Criminal Justice in France in the Nineteenth and Twentieth Centuries* (University of North Carolina Press, 2010), 12.

2. Femme Fiquet, 9th interrogation, 19 July 1882. Marie Fenet statement (given in Dole), 15 July 1882.

3. Karen E. Carter, *Scandal in the Parish: Priests and Parishioners Behaving Badly in Eighteenth-Century France* (McGill-Queen's University Press, 2019).

4. In two subfolders, "Lettres Affaire Fiquet" and "Lettres de l'Abbé Pihéry."

5. François (l'Abbé) Pihéry statement, 15 July 1882.

6. "Commission rogatoire," Dijon examining magistrate to the Besançon examining magistrate, 29 July 1882. The note does not tell us any more about who these people were and why they were contacted. We can infer from the note that the incident had been mentioned by Fenet.

7. Letter from the Abbé Pihéry to the femme Fiquet, 7 July 1879.

8. Marie Fenet statement (given in Dole, Jura), 15 July 1882.

9. See chap. 5 for the discussion of this incident during the trial.

10. Marie Fenet statement (given in Dole), 15 July 1882.

11. Note from the examining magistrate, Alfred Loiseau, to the procureur, 28 October 1882, forwarding a note from the Tribunal d'instance de Dole confirming the birth dates of the two girls.

12. Harris, *Murders and Madness*, 126.

13. Kalifa gives several journalistic examples from the turn of the century where concern is expressed about the motives of women testifying in serious cases. See "Les femmes, le crime et l'enquête," in *Femmes et justice pénale, XIXᵉ–XXᵉ siècles*, ed. Christine Bard et al. (Presses universitaires de Rennes, 2002), 283–92.

14. Gide also noted two cases of child molestation by fathers where the sentence was lenient because the juries considered the mothers' evidence unreliable. See chaps. 3 and 5 of "Souvenirs de la Cour d'assises," in Gide, *Ne jugez pas*.

15. See Fuchs, *Poor and Pregnant in Paris*.

16. Nejma Omari, "Que toute femme choisisse elle-même sa destinée! Le droit à l'avortement avant la loi Veil," BNF Gallica blog, 15 January 2021. https://gallica.bnf.fr/blog/15012021/que-toute-femme-choisisse-elle-meme-sa-destinee-le-droit-lavortement-avant-la-loi-veil?mode=desktop#block-commentsblock-comment-form-block.

17. René Le Mée, "Une affaire de 'faiseuses d'anges' à la fin du XIXᵉ siècle," *Communications* (1986): 137–74, 140.

18. Le Mée, "Une affaire de 'faiseuse d'anges,'" 142–43.

19. Veuve Barbey statement, 8 July 1882.

20. Marandon, "De la morphinomanie," 670.

21. Michelot's statement, given in Paris on 22 July 1882, refers to Fiquet as "une hystérique" with "des idées romanesques."

22. For an extended discussion of such monomanias, see Laure Murat, *The Man Who Thought He Was Napoleon: Toward a Political History of Madness* (University of Chicago Press, 2014).

23. Marie Cagnard statement, 8 July 1882.

24. Dr. Gautrelet statement, 28 July 1882; Madeleine Garnier statement, 28 July 1882.

25. "Affaire Fiquet," *La Côte d'Or*, 3 July 1882.

26. Note from examining magistrate, Alfred Loiseau, to the procureur, 28 October 1882, forwarding a note from the Tribunal d'instance de Dole confirming birth dates of the two girls.

27. Marie Cagnard statement, 8 July 1882.

28. Marie Bautut statement, 10 July 1882.

29. Lombroso, *Female Offender*, 213–14, 247–52.

30. This is a point made in the introduction to Donovan, *Juries and the Transformation of Criminal Justice in France.*

31. Harris, *Murders and Madness*, 36–37. The case was reported in the *Gazette des Tribunaux*, 26 June 1897.

32. Barbara Ehrenreich and Deirdre English, *Witches, Midwives and Nurses: A History of Women Healers* (Writers and Readers Publishing Cooperative, 1976), 1–25.

33. For further discussion of population decline, see Brunelle and Finley-Croswhite, *Murder in the Métro*, 70–71, and Nimisha Barton, *Reproductive Citizens: Gender, Immigration, and the State in Modern France, 1880–1945* (Cornell University Press, 2021).

34. Hannah Frydman, "Freedom's Sex Problem: Classified Advertising, Law, and the Politics of Reading in Third Republic France," *French Historical Studies* 44, no. 4 (2021): 688.

35. Femme Fiquet, 9th and 19th interrogations, 19 July 1882 and 26 October 1882.

36. Louise Fiquet statement, 4 July 1882.

37. Louise Fiquet statement, 20 October 1882.

38. Claude Coupé statement, 26 October 1882.

39. Note no. 43, "procès-verbal police."

40. Letter from the Femme Fiquet to Loiseau, 22 October 1882.

41. *Gazette des Tribunaux*, 14 September 1867.

42. Ruth Ellen Homrighaus, "Baby Farming: The Care of Illegitimate Children in England, 1860–1943," PhD diss., University of North Carolina at Chapel Hill, 2003, 1–2.

43. Homrighaus, "Baby Farming," iii.

44. Homrighaus, "Baby Farming," 3–6.

45. Homrighaus, "Baby Farming," 34–51, 52, 69–70.

46. This statement is related only in an undated request for information from Alfred Loiseau to the Besançon *juge de paix*, sent during the early stages of the investigation.

47. "Cour d'assises de la Côte-d'Or: Une petite fille de six ans noyée dans le canal de Dijon," *Le Figaro*, 9 March 1883.

48. Pierre Fiquet, 1st interrogation.

49. Deroye statement, 6 July 1882.

50. Louise Fiquet statement, 4 July 1882.

51. Elizabeth Yardley and David Wilson, "In Search of the 'Angels of Death': Conceptualising the Contemporary Nurse Healthcare Serial Killer," *Journal of Investigative Psychology and Offender Profiling* 13, no. 1 (2016): 39–55.

52. Béla Bodó, "The Poisoning Women of Tiszazug," *Journal of Family History* 27, no. 1 (2002): 40–59. The story is told in greater detail in Bodó's monograph: *Tiszazug: A Social History of a Murder Epidemic* (East European Monographs, 2002). It is effectively dramatized in Patti McCracken's fictional version of the story, *The Angel Makers: The True Story of the Most Astonishing Murder Ring in History* (Mudlark, 2023).

53. See, for example, the *Observer*, 8 September 1929.

54. On the 1845 poisons law, see Jean-Jacques Yvorel, "De la loi 'Lafarge' à la loi de 1916: Aux origines de la pénalisation des stupéfiants," *Psychotropes* 23, no. 2 (2016): 11–23.

55. See chap. 2 of Downing, *Subject of Murder*, and chap. 1 of Hartman, *Victorian Murderesses*, on the Lafarge poisoning affair.

56. Lisa Downing, "Murder in the Feminine: Marie Lafarge and the Sexualization of the Nineteenth-Century Criminal Woman," *Journal of the History of Sexuality* 18, no. 1 (2009): 124.

57. Michelle Perrot, "Ouverture," in *Femmes et justice pénale: XIXᵉ–XXᵉ siècles*, ed. Christine Bard et al. (Presses universitaires de Rennes, 2002), 9–21.

58. "Affaire Fiquet," *La Démocratie Bourguignonne*, 8 March 1883.

59. Letter from the mayor of Moissey to the femme Fiquet.

60. Femme Fiquet, 3rd interrogation.

4. The Medical Reports

1. Harris, *Murders and Madness*, 1–2; on the role of medico-legists, see also 146–47.

2. Dr. Blanche, "Procès de la femme Fiquet (De Dijon) accusée d'assassinat, morphinomanie et simulation: Rapport médico-légal." *Annales médico-psychologiques*, no. 10 (1883): 240. The asylum, a former monastery, is also sometimes called "l'asile des Chartreux."

3. Marandon, "De la morphinomanie," 695.

4. Harris, *Murders and Madness*, 2.

5. See "Les débuts de la psychiatrie dans les hôpitaux généraux de l'Assistance publique de Paris," *Psychiatrie, Sciences humaines, Neurosciences* 10, no. 2 (2012): 95–101.

6. See Jessie Hewitt, *Institutionalizing Gender: Madness, the Family, and Psychiatric Power in Nineteenth-Century France* (Cornell University Press, 2020), 158–62. Hewitt bases her observations on Marandon de Montyel, "La nouvelle hospitalization des aliénés par la method de liberté et son application en Ville-Évrard," *Annales médico-psychologiques* 3 (1896): 65, and "Des asiles d'aliénés à portes ouvertes (suite)," *Annales médico-psychologiques* 6 (1897): 275–81.

7. Hewitt, *Institutionalizing Gender*, 163.

8. Joseph, *Unlawful Killings*, 49.

9. Marandon, "De la morphinomanie," 667.

10. Marandon, "De la morphinomanie," 705.

11. The German doctor Levinstein first published on the problem of the morphine habit in 1877, *Die Morphiumsucht*, translated into English as *Morbid Craving*

for Morphia (Smith, Elder, 1878). Although the problem of morphine dependency was known, it was not until the later 1880s and early 1890s that a wider literature in French would be available to investigating doctors like Marandon.

12. Marandon, "De la morphinomanie," 702.

13. See Michael Finn, *Figures of the Pre-Freudian Unconscious* (Cambridge University Press, 2017), 131. In opposition to Charcot's view were the experts of the Nancy school, who asserted a different opinion on the nature and power of unconscious activity. See Ruth Harris, "Murder Under Hypnosis," *Psychological Medicine* 15, no. 3 (1985): 477–505.

14. "The Trial of Michel Eyraud and Gabrielle Bompard," *Spectator*, 20 December 1890, 891.

15. Artières, "Crimes écrits," 48–61.

16. Philippe Artières, *Un séminariste assassin: L'affaire Bladier, 1905* (CNRS Editions, 2020), 38–39.

17. Downing, *Subject of Murder*, 69; Ryckère, *La Femme en prison*, 84.

18. See chap. 7 of Gide, "Souvenirs de la Cour d'Assises." It discusses "L'affaire Charles," the case of a jealous man who stabbed his lover at least 110 times in front of a neighbor, and the Redureau affair (Gide, *Ne jugez pas*, 51–59, 97–121).

19. Marandon, "De la morphinomanie," 667–70.

20. Marandon, "De la morphinomanie," 671.

21. Marandon, "De la morphinomanie," 669.

22. Bénédict Augustin Morel, *Traité des dégénérescences physiques, intellectuelles et morales de l'espèce humaine* (Baillière, 1857), cited in Marandon, "De la morphinomanie," 672.

23. On female prostitution as an industry / economy and its crossover with working-class occupations in the nineteenth century, see Corbin, *Les Filles de noce*.

24. See Fuchs, *Poor and Pregnant in Paris*, 9.

25. Marandon, "De la morphinomanie," 668–69.

26. Marandon, "De la morphinomanie," 673.

27. Marandon, "De la morphinomanie," 679.

28. See Black, "Morphine on Trial," 628–30.

29. According to Blanche ("Procès de la femme Fiquet," 251). Not all these testimonies were recorded in the press reports.

30. All citations in this paragraph are from Marandon, "De la morphinomanie," 669.

31. Marandon, "De la morphinomanie," 670. On the dose, see also Blanche, "Procès de la femme Fiquet," 237.

32. Marandon, "De la morphinomanie," 676.

33. Marandon, "De la morphinomanie," 679.

34. Marandon, "De la morphinomanie," 673–74, citing Levinstein, *Die Morphiumsucht*.

35. Marandon, "De la morphinomanie," 687. Marandon claimed to be citing Levinstein, Lunier, Brouardel, and Hallez in this section (all emerging experts in the field of morphine addiction), although he does not give full references.

36. Marandon, "De la morphinomanie," 689–90.

37. Marandon, "De la morphinomanie," 691.

38. Marandon, "De la morphinomanie," 690.

39. Marandon, "De la morphinomanie," 683.

40. Marandon, "De la morphinomanie," 687.

41. Some doctors wrote about their own (and their colleagues') experimentation with morphine and subsequent addiction. See Ernest Chambard, *La Morphinomanie* (Reuff, 1890), and Georges Pichon, *Le Morphinisme* (O. Doin, 1889).

42. Marandon, "De la morphinomanie," 671.

43. Marandon, "De la morphinomanie," 693.

44. Marandon, "De la morphinomanie," 669.

45. Norris, *L'écriture du défi*, 107–9.

46. Marandon, "De la morphinomanie," 673–74.

47. Marandon, "De la morphinomanie," 675.

48. Marandon, "De la morphinomanie," 680.

49. Marandon, "De la morphinomanie," 684–85.

50. Marandon, "De la morphinomanie," 697. Emphasis in original.

51. Brady Brower, *Unruly Spirits*, xxiii.

52. See Nicole Edelman, *Voyantes, guérisseuses et visionnaires en France: 1785–1914* (Albin Michel, 1995).

53. Marandon, "De la morphinomanie," 697–98.

54. Marandon, "De la morphinomanie," 700–701.

55. Marandon, "De la morphinomanie," 703.

56. Downing, *Subject of Murder*, 13.

57. Jan Goldstein, *Console and Classify: The French Psychiatric Profession in the Nineteenth Century* (Cambridge University Press, 1987), 326.

58. See Jonathan W. Marshall, *Performing Neurology: The Dramaturgy of Dr. Jean-Martin Charcot* (Palgrave Macmillan, 2016).

59. Thibaut Maus de Rolley, *Moi, Louis Gaufridy, ayant soufflé plus de mille femmes: Une confession de sorcier au XVIIe siècle* (Belles Lettres, 2023), 9.

60. Maus de Rolley, *Moi, Louis Gaufridy*, 9.

61. Marandon, "De la morphinomanie," 702.

62. Marandon, "De la morphinomanie," 702.

63. Blanche, "Procès de la femme Fiquet," 235.

64. "Affaire Fiquet," *Le Progrès de la Côte-d'Or*, 5 March 1883.

65. Marandon, "De la morphinomanie," 678.

66. René Semelaigne, *Les pionniers de la psychiatrie française avant et après Pinel* (Baillière, 1930), 70–71. Semelaigne, who was the grandson of the nineteenth-century pioneer Casimir Pinel, provides a detailed intellectual biography of the principal figures in alienist medicine. See also Jan Goldstein, *Console and Classify*, 392. On the clinic founded by Esprit Blanche in 1821, see Laure Murat, *La maison du docteur Blanche: Histoire d'un asile et de ses pensionnaires, de Nerval à Maupassant* (Lattès, 2001).

67. Harris, *Murders and Madness*, 146–47.

68. On the vie de famille approach, see Jessie Hewitt, *Institutionalizing Gender: Madness, the Family, and Psychiatric Power in Nineteenth-Century France* (Cornell University Press, 2020), 69–77.

69. Blanche, "Procès de la femme Fiquet," 236–37.

70. Blanche, "Procès de la femme Fiquet," 237–39.

71. Blanche, "Procès de la femme Fiquet," 235.

72. Blanche, "Procès de la femme Fiquet," 241–42.

73. Blanche, "Procès de la femme Fiquet," 242.

74. Blanche, "Procès de la femme Fiquet," 242.

75. The Petit Robert dictionary gives the synonyms *écraser, abattre, opprimer, fatiguer, excéder, accuser,* and the Robert Collins dictionary gives the English translation "to overwhelm, to overcome" as well as "to condemn, to damn." It is interesting that *condamner* is not given as a French synonym, suggesting that the verb *accabler* in this context is better translated as "to damn," as in "a damning piece of evidence."

76. Blanche, "Procès de la femme Fiquet," 242.

77. Blanche, "Procès de la femme Fiquet," 243.

78. Blanche, "Procès de la femme Fiquet," 243–45.

79. Philippe Artières, "Un séminariste assassin."

80. Philippe Artières, "Crimes écrits," 58–59.

81. Artières, "Crimes écrits," 240.

82. See chap. 3 of Downing, *Subject of Murder,* for a discussion of sexual murder as a perversion of the reproductive instinct. The idea was originally outlined by Krafft-Ebing in *Psychopathia Sexualis: The Case Histories* (F. A. Davis, 1892).

83. Blanche, "Procès de la femme Fiquet," 246.

84. Blanche, "Procès de la femme Fiquet," 247.

85. Blanche, "Procès de la femme Fiquet," 247–48.

86. Brady Brower, *Unruly Spirits,* xv–xviii.

87. Brady Brower, *Unruly Spirits,* xviii.

88. Henri F. Ellenberger, *The Discovery of the Unconscious: The History and Evolution of Dynamic Psychiatry* (Basic, 1970).

89. See Charles Richet, *Traité de métapsychique* (Alcan, 1922). Cited in Brady Brower, *Unruly Spirits,* xvii.

90. Brady Brower, *Unruly Spirits,* xix.

91. Blanche, "Procès de la femme Fiquet," 249–51.

92. Blanche, "Procès de la femme Fiquet," 253.

93. Blanche, "Procès de la femme Fiquet," 249.

Interlude

1. See Corbin, *Les filles de noce,* for a discussion of the idea of the working classes as a metaphorical valve, sewer, or outlet promoted by social hygiene specialists such as Alexandre Parent-Duchâtelet.

2. Karine Salomé, "Voleur ou assassin? Discours et représentations autour de l'affaire Troppmann (1869–1870)," in *Au Voleur!,* ed. Frédéric Chauvaud and Arnaud-Dominique Houte (Éditions de la Sorbonne, 2014), 119.

3. Perrot, "L'affaire Troppmann (1869)," 28–31.

4. Perrot, "L'affaire Troppmann (1869)," 32.

5. Perrot, "L'affaire Troppmann (1869)," 30.

6. Fuchs, *Poor and Pregnant in Paris,* 35–36.

7. Perrot, "L'affaire Troppmann (1869)," 30.

8. Athanäse Barbey's conviction was reported in *Le Gaulois,* 22 August 1883. Marandon also called the Barbey family "people without morals" in his report (see Marandon, "De la morphinomanie," 701).

9. Perrot, "L'affaire Troppmann (1869)," 34.

10. Zemon Davis, *Return of Martin Guerre*, 22.

11. Artières, "Crimes Écrits," 55.

12. Artières, *Un séminariste assassin*, 40.

13. *Le Rappel*, 4 January 1870. Cited in Perrot, "L'affaire Troppmann," 36.

14. Gelfand, *Imagination in Confinement*, 42–43.

15. Le Mée, "Une affaire de 'faiseuses d'anges,'" 141.

16. Ryckère, *La femme en prison*, 160–89.

17. Le Mée, "Une affaire de 'faiseuses d'anges,'" 143–47.

18. Gelfand, *Imagination in Confinement*, 43.

19. Le Mée, "Une affaire de 'faiseuses d'anges,'" 155.

20. Le Mée, "Une affaire de 'faiseuses d'anges,'" 155.

21. Artières, *Un séminariste assassin*, citing Dr. Moll, *Les perversions de l'instinct génital* (Carré, 1893).

22. Ernest Dupré, *Les empoisonneurs: Étude historique, psychologique et médico-légale* (A. Rey, 1909), 7.

23. Perrot, "L'affaire Troppmann (1869)," 37. On the male murderer as genius, see also Downing's discussion of Lacenaire in *Subject of Murder*.

24. Perrot, "L'affaire Troppmann (1869)," 32–33.

25. Perrot, "L'affaire Troppmann (1869)," 34–35.

26. Salomé, "Voleur ou assassin?," 30.

27. Salomé, "Voleur ou assassin?," 37–44.

5. The Trial

1. These details are taken from the genealogy website Geneanet: https://gw.geneanet.org/lpinon1?lang=fr&pz=laurent&nz=pinon&p=etienne&n=metman. I also obtained a copy of the eulogy given at Metman's funeral on a personal family web page here, but the page no longer exists: http://nadine-emmanuel.clause.pagesperso-orange.fr/famille/emetman/index.html.

2. V. Wright, É. Anceau, and S. Hazareesingh, *Les Préfets de Gambetta* (Presses de l'université Paris-Sorbonne, 2007).

3. Mairet's first name is not given in the press reports or trial documentation.

4. "Affaire Fiquet," *La Démocratie Bourguignonne*, 6 March 1883.

5. Donovan, *Juries and the Transformation of Criminal Justice in France*, 12.

6. All details of the trial cited here are taken from coverage in *La Démocratie Bourguignonne* of 6, 7, and 8 March 1883 (unless otherwise indicated).

7. Robert A. Nye, *Crime, Madness, & Politics in Modern France: The Medical Concept of National Decline* (Princeton University Press, 1984), 18–20.

8. Foucault, *Moi, Pierre Rivière*, 270–71.

9. Kalifa, "Les femmes, le crime et l'enquête," 283–92.

10. Donovan, *Juries and the Transformation of Criminal Justice in France*.

11. Berenson, *Trial of Madame Caillaux*, 6, 15. See also chap. 6 of this book on the role of the press in the Caillaux trial.

12. See Guillais, *Crimes of Passion*, 182–83, on the typology of crimes of passion.

13. Foucault, *Moi, Pierre Rivière*, 271.

14. As Norris notes, Lombroso's ideas were widely challenged by other criminologists and anthropologists, such as Alexandre Lacassagne, Gabriel Tarde, and Henry Joly, who would propose social theories of criminality. See Norris, *L'Écriture du défi*, 104–5.

15. Brunelle and Finley-Croswhite, *Murder in the Métro*, 60.

16. "Assises de la Côte-d'Or," *Le Droit Populaire*, 6 March 1883. Much the same account was given in *La Démocratie Bourguignonne*.

17. "Assises de la Côte-d'Or," *Le Figaro*, 9 March 1883. Curiously, this event was reported in the national press but not in the more detailed regional reports. It was not mentioned by Dr. Blanche, the last medical professional to examine the femme Fiquet.

18. Kalifa, "Les Femmes, le crime et l'enquête," para. 1–12 (unpaginated online ed). See also Philippe Artières and Dominique Kalifa, *Vidal, le tueur de femmes: Une biographie sociale* (Verdier, 2017).

19. "Déposition de M. Le Docteur Weil," *La Démocratie Bourguignonne*, 7 March 1883. The doctor called her "une farceuse et une comédienne."

20. "Affaire Fiquet," *La Démocratie Bourguignonne*, 6 March 1883. The journalist is referring to the original trial date in December 1882.

21. "Affaire Fiquet," *Le Progrès*, 5 March 1883. The same words were reported in *La Côte-d'Or* on 6 March 1883.

22. On the typology of the born criminal versus the "passionate" criminal, see Guillais, *Crimes of Passion*, 183.

23. "Affaire Fiquet," *Le Bien Public*, 6 March 1883.

24. "Assises de la Côte-d'Or," *Le Figaro*, 9 March 1883.

25. "Affaire Fiquet," *La Démocratie Bourguignonne*, 6 March 1883.

26. "Affaire Fiquet," *La Démocratie Bourguignonne*, 6 March 1883.

27. "Affaire Fiquet," *La Démocratie Bourguignonne*, 6 March 1883.

28. "Affaire Fiquet," *La Démocratie Bourguignonne*, 6 March 1883.

29. "Affaire Fiquet," *La Démocratie Bourguignonne*, 6 March 1883.

30. "Affaire Fiquet," *La Démocratie Bourguignonne*, 6 March 1883.

31. "Affaire Fiquet," *La Démocratie Bourguignonne*, 7 March 1883.

32. "Affaire Fiquet," *La Démocratie Bourguignonne*, 6–7 March 1883.

33. Harris, *Murders and Madness*, 21.

34. "Déposition de Madame la Veuve Barbey," *La Démocratie Bourguignonne*, 7 March 1883.

35. "Déposition de Marie Gagnard" [*sic*]. *La Démocratie Bourguignonne*, 7 March 1883.

36. See, for example, Dumas (fils), *Les femmes qui tuent et les femmes qui votent* (C. Lévy, 1880), which contains several anecdotal examples of men who went unpunished for their moral misdeameanours, leading to women taking the law into their own hands.

37. "Déposition de Marie Fenet," *La Démocratie Bourguignonne*, 8 March 1883.

38. "Affaire Fiquet," *La Démocratie Bourguignonne*, 8 March 1883.

39. "Déposition de Madame Lefebvre," *La Démocratie Bourguignonne*, 7 March 1883.

40. "Déposition de Madame Lefebvre," *La Démocratie Bourguignonne*, 7 March 1883.

41. "Affaire Fiquet," *La Démocratie Bourguignonne*, 8 March 1883.

42. "Affaire Fiquet," *La Démocratie Bourguignonne*, 7–8 March 1883.

43. Ferguson, *Gender and Justice*, 7.

44. "Affaire Fiquet," *La Démocratie Bourguignonne*, 7 March 1883.

45. "Affaire Fiquet," *La Démocratie Bourgignonne*, 8 March 1883.

46. Gide, *Ne jugez pas*, 42.

47. See Black, "Morphine on Trial," showing that the Aubert case was cited in full (transcript). The Fiquet affair does not feature in the 1883 *Gazette*.

48. "Affaire Fiquet," *La Démocratie Bourguignonne*, 8 March 1883. *Le Catholique*, 10 March 1883.

49. "Affaire Fiquet," *La Démocratie Bourguignonne*, 8 March 1883.

50. "Réquisitoire de M. L'avocat général" (Mairet), *La Démocratie Bourguignonne*, 8 March 1883.

51. "Affaire Fiquet," *La Démocratie Bourguignonne*, 8 March 1883.

52. "Affaire Fiquet," *La Démocratie Bourguignonne*, 8 March 1883.

53. Maza, *Violette Nozière*, 188.

54. "Plaidoirie de M. Metman," *La Démocratie Bourguignonne*, 8 March 1883.

55. Donovan, *Juries and the Transformation of Criminal Justice in France*, 13–14.

56. On the introduction of "circonstances atténuantes" in the 1832 reform of the French penal code, see Guillais, *Crimes of Passion*, 172.

57. Donovan, *Juries and the Transformation of Criminal Justice in France*, 17–18.

58. "Affaire Fiquet," *La Côte-d'Or*, 9 March 1883.

6. Afterlives

1. This statistic accounts for high infant mortality rates and records how long women who survived to adulthood could expect to live. Institut national d'études démographiques (INED): https://www.ined.fr/fr/tout-savoir-population /graphiques-cartes/graphiques-interpretes/esperance-vie-france/.

2. Louise Michel, *Le Livre du bagne*, ed. Véronique Fau-Vincenti (Presses universitaires de Lyon, 2001). Cited in Nancy Sloan Goldberg, "The Radicalization of Louise Michel," in *Prison Narratives from Boethius to Zana*, ed. Philip E. Phillips (Palgrave Macmillan, 2014), 125–26.

3. Odile Krakovitch, *Les femmes bagnardes* (O. Orban, 1990), 9–12.

4. Odile Krakovitch, email message to author, 17 October 2024.

5. The Fiquet case is cited in Chambard, *La morphinomanie*, 170; Léopold Ducasse, "Contribution à l'étude de la morphine et de l'intoxication par cet alcaloïde," (PhD diss., Montpellier, 1887), 56–61; Henri Guimbail, "Crimes et délits commis par les morphinomanes," *Annales d'hygiène publique et de médecine légale* 3 (1891): 481–501.

6. Black, "Morphine on Trial," 629.

7. Black, "Morphine on Trial," 639, 650.

8. Henri Guimbail, *Les morphinomanes* (Baillière, 1892), 221–28.

9. Guimbail, *Les morphinomanes*, 227–29.

10. Veuve Tissot, letter to the examining magistrate (Loiseau), 11 July 1882.

11. On Athanäse Barbey's conviction, see *Le Gaulois*, 22 August 1883. Marandon, "De la morphinomanie," 701.

12. ADCO, 2 U 1495. "Liasse supplémentaire" (a folder containing supplementary evidence relating to Marie-Françoise Fiquet's trial). Statements from Justine

Jobard and Maria Jobard, and Sœur Clotilde Marie, 2 March 1883. It seems this evidence was gathered too late to be included in the trial proceedings.

13. Letter dated 22 February 1883 from the railway board to the examining magistrate, confirming that Fiquet had been at work at the station on 10 April 1882.

14. "Special Correspondence," *British Medical Journal* 8 (1895): 1301, https://doi.org/10.1136/bmj.1.1797.1301.

15. Harris, *Murders and Madness*, 27. Dr. Blanche, however, was at the end of his career, and he died in 1893 at the age of seventy-two. His last publication was a commissioned report on asylum reform that came out in 1884, a year after the Fiquet trial: Émile Blanche, *Rapport à l'Académie de Médecine sur les projets de réforme relatifs à la législation sur les aliénés* (Masson, 1884).

16. "Special Correspondence," *British Medical Journal* 25 (1896): 240, https://doi.org/10.1136/bmj.1.1830.240.

17. Marandon de Montyel, *Le nouvel asile d'aliénés de la Seine et les asiles unisexués* (G. Maurin, 1895), 15.

18. Marandon de Montyel, "Obsessions et impulsions," *Archives de l'anthropologie criminelle (1886–1914)* 19 (1904): 81–126.

19. Marandon, "Obsessions et impulsions," 81–82.

20. Marandon, "Obsessions et impulsions," 116–17.

21. Marandon's ideas would also be developed in a later text, in which he partially rejected Freud's claim of the sexual origin of all obsessions. Marandon argued that many obsessions arise in adolescence. See Marandon de Montyel, *Obsessions et vie sexuelle* (Imprimerie de Charles Hérissey, 1905), 291.

22. Marandon de Montyel, "Contribution à l'étude des aliénés poursuivis, condamnés et acquittés," *Archives de l'anthropologie criminelle* 15 (1900): 401–18.

23. Susannah Wilson, "To Whom Does a Letter Belong? Psychopathology and Epistolography in the Asylum Letters of Antonin Artaud and Camille Claudel," *Modern Languages Open*, 1 (2021): 1–18; Antonin Artaud, *Lettres: 1937–1943* (Paris: Gallimard, 2015); Camille Claudel, *Correspondance*, Anne Rivière and Bruno Gaudichon (eds.) (Gallimard, 2014); André Roumieux, *Artaud et l'asile* (Séguier, 1996).

24. Repper, "Munchausen Syndrome by Proxy in Health Care Workers," 302.

25. Robert Jay Lifton, *The Nazi Doctors: Medical Killing and the Psychology of Genocide* (Macmillan, 1986), 5. In his conceptual framing, Lifton owed much to Hannah Arendt's concept of the "banality of evil" as originally outlined in 1963 in *Eichmann in Jerusalem: A Report on the Banality of Evil* (Penguin, 1994).

26. Lifton, *Nazi Doctors*, 47, 60.

27. Krakovitch, *Les femmes bagnardes*, 12.

BIBLIOGRAPHY

Archives

Archives Départementales de la Côte-d'Or (ADCO):
>   2 U 1333—Cours d'appel et d'assises, mag. M tr. 123, ta. 2, case number 8, 7
>   March 1883
>   2 U 1495—the *dossier de procédure* for the Fiquet prosecution case

Primary Sources

d'Almond, Comte. *Six années de morphinomanie*. Éditions du livre moderne, 1910.

Blanche, Dr. "Procès de la femme Fiquet (de Dijon), accusée d'assassinat, morphinomanie et simulation. Rapport médico-légal." *Annales médico-psychologiques*, no. 10 (1883): 234–53.

Blanche, Émile. *Rapport à l'Académie de Médecine sur les projets de réforme relatifs à la législation sur les aliénés*. Masson, 1884.

Boisseau, Edmond. *Des maladies simulées et des moyens de les reconnaître*. Baillière, 1870.

Chabeuf, Henri. *Dijon à travers les âges: Histoire et description*. Damidot Frères, 1897.

Chambard, Ernest. *La morphinomanie: Étude clinique, médico-légale et thérapeutique*. Reuff, 1890.

Charcot, M. Le Professeur. *Clinique des maladies du système nerveux (1889–90)*. Progrès médical, 1890.

Chavigny, Paul. *Diagnostique des maladies simulées dans les accidents du travail et devant les Conseils de révision et de réforme de l'armée et de la marine*. Baillière, 1906.

Derblich, Wolfgang. *Des maladies simulées dans l'armée et des moyens de les reconnaître*. Translated (from German to French) by Adrien Schmit. Asselin, 1883.

Ducasse, Léopold. "Contribution à l'étude de la morphine et de l'intoxication par cet alcaloïde." PhD diss., Montpellier, 1887.

Dumas (fils), Alexandre. *Les femmes qui tuent et les femmes qui votent*. C. Lévy, 1880.

Dupré, Ernest. *Les empoisonneurs: Étude historique psychologique et médico-légale*. A. Rey, 1909.

Fodéreé, F. E. *Essai médico-légal sur les diverses espèces de folie vraie, simulée et raisonnée*. L. F. Le Roux, 1832.

Gavin, Hector. *On Feigned and Factitious Diseases*. J. Churchill, 1843.

Granier, Camille. *La femme criminelle*. O. Doin, 1906.

Guimbail, Henri. "Crimes et délits commis par les morphinomanes." *Annales d'hygiène publique et de médecine légale* 3, no. 25 (1891): 481–572.

Guimbail, Henri. *Les morphinomanes*. J.-B. Baillière et fils, 1892.

Huguet, J. *Recherches sur les maladies simulées et mutilations volontaires*. H. Charles-Lavauzelle, 1900.

Levinstein, *Die Morphiumsucht* (translated into English as *Morbid Craving for Morphia*, 1878). Smith, Elder, 1878.

Lombroso, Cesare, and William Ferrero. *The Female Offender*. Appleton, 1900.

Marandon de Montyel, Évariste. "Contribution à l'étude des aliénés poursuivis, condamnés et acquittés." *Archives de l'anthropologie criminelle* 15 (1900): 401–18.

Marandon de Montyel, Evariste. "De la morphinomanie dans ses rapports avec la médecine légale." *L'Encéphale. Journal des maladies mentales et nerveuses* 3, no. 1 (1883): 667–706.

Marandon de Montyel, Évariste. "Des asiles d'aliénés à portes ouvertes (suite)." *Annales médico-psychologiques* 6 (1897): 275–81.

Marandon de Montyel, Évariste. "La Nouvelle hospitalisation des aliénés par la méthode de liberté et son application en Ville-Évrard." *Annales médico-psychologiques* 3 (1896): 65.

Marandon de Montyel, Évariste. *Le nouvel asile d'aliénés de la Seine et les asiles unisexués*. Imprimerie de G. Maurin, 1895.

Marandon de Montyel, Évariste. "Obsessions et impulsions." *Archives de l'anthropologie criminelle (1886–1914)* 19 (1904): 81–126.

Marandon de Montyel, Evariste. *Obsessions et vie sexuelle*. Imprimerie de Charles Hérissey, 1905.

"The Medical Work in Hospitals for the Insane." *Journal of the American Medical Association* 42, no. 12 (1904): 770–71.

Menninger, Karl A. "Psychology of a Certain Type of Malingering." *Archives of Neurology and Psychiatry* 33 (1935): 507–15.

Moll, Dr. Albert. *Les perversions de l'instinct génital*. Carré, 1893.

Morel, Bénédict Augustin. *Traité des dégénérescences physiques, intellectuelles et morales de l'espèce humaine et des causes qui produisent ces variétés maladives*. J. B. Baillière, 1857.

Pichon, Georges. *Le morphinisme: Impulsions délictueuses, troubles physiques et mentaux des morphinomanes, leur capacité et leur situation juridique*. O. Doin, 1889.

Régnier, Dr. Louis Raoul. *L'intoxication chronique par la morphine et ses diverses formes*. Progrès Médical, 1890.

Ryckère, Raymond de. *La femme en prison et devant la mort: Étude de criminologie*. A. Storck, 1898.

Saussay, Victorien du. *La Morphine: roman passionnel*. A. Méricant, 1906.

Schwaeblé, René. *Les Voluptés de la morphine*. Bibliothèque de l'inconnu, 1908.

Secondary Sources

Anon. "Les débuts de la psychiatrie dans les hôpitaux généraux de l'Assistance publique de Paris." *Psychiatrie, Sciences humaines, Neurosciences* 10, no. 2 (2012): 95–101.

American Psychiatric Association, *Diagnostic and Statistical Manual of Mental Disorders*, 5th ed., 2013.

Arendt, Hannah. *Eichmann in Jerusalem: A Report on the Banality of Evil*. Penguin, 1994.

Arnold, John H. "The Historian as Inquisitor: The Ethics of Interrogating Subaltern Voices." *Rethinking History* 2, no. 3 (1998): 379–86.

Artaud, Antonin. *Lettres: 1937–1943*. Gallimard, 2015.

Artières, Philippe. "Crimes écrits: La collection d'autobiographies de criminels du Professeur A. Lacassagne." *Genèses: Sciences Sociales et Histoire*, 1995, 48–67.

Artières, Philippe. *Un séminariste assassin. L'affaire Bladier, 1905*. CNRS Editions, 2020.

Artières, Philippe, and Dominique Kalifa. *Vidal, le tueur de femmes: Une biographie sociale*. Verdier, 2017.

Asher, Richard. "Munchausen's Syndrome." *Lancet* 257, no. 6650 (1951): 339–41.

Bard, Christine, Frédéric Chauvaud, Michelle Perrot, and Jacques-Guy Petit, eds. *Femmes et justice pénale: XIXᵉ–XXᵉ siècles*. Presses universitaires de Rennes, 2002.

Barton, Nimisha. *Reproductive Citizens: Gender, Immigration, and the State in Modern France, 1880–1945*. Cornell University Press, 2021.

Berenson, Edward. *The Trial of Madame Caillaux*. University of California Press, 1992.

Bernheimer, Charles. *Figures of Ill Repute: Representing Prostitution in Nineteenth-Century France*. Duke University Press, 1997.

Berridge, Virginia. *Opium and the People: Opiate Use and Policy in Nineteenth and Early Twentieth Century England*. Free Association, 1999.

Black, Sara E. "Morphine on Trial: Legal Medicine and Criminal Responsibility in the Fin-de-Siècle." *French Historical Studies* 42, no. 4 (2019): 623–53. https://doi.org/10.1215/00161071-7689198.

Bodó, Béla. "The Poisoning Women of Tiszazug." *Journal of Family History* 27, no. 1 (2002): 40–59. https://doi.org/10.1177/036319900202700103.

Bodó, Béla. *Tiszazug: A Social History of a Murder Epidemic*. East European Monographs, 2002.

Botbol, Michel, and Adeline Gourbil. "The Place of Psychoanalysis in French Psychiatry." *BJPsych International* 15, no. 1 (2018): 3–5. https://doi.org/10.1192/bji.2017.3.

Brady Brower, M. *Unruly Spirits: The Science of Psychic Phenomena in Modern France*. University of Illinois Press, 2010.

Breuer, Josef, and Sigmund Freud. *Studies on Hysteria*. Vol. 2 of *The Standard Edition of the Complete Psychological Works of Sigmund Freud*, edited and translated by J. Strachey et al. Hogarth, 1893–95.

Briggs, Jonathyne. "From Collaboration to Resistance: The Family Dynamic in Autism Literature in Contemporary France." *Contemporary European History* 32, no. 2 (2023): 254–69.

Brunelle, Gayle K., and Annette Finley-Croswhite. *Murder in the Métro: Lætitia Toureaux and the Cagoule in 1930s France*. Louisiana State University Press, 2010.

Capote, Truman. *In Cold Blood: A True Account of a Multiple Murder and Its Consequences*. Random House, 1965.

Carter, Karen E. *Scandal in the Parish: Priests and Parishioners Behaving Badly in Eighteenth-Century France*. McGill-Queen's University Press, 2019.

Caruth, Cathy. *Unclaimed Experience: Trauma, Narrative, and History*. Johns Hopkins University Press, 2007.

Chevalier, Louis. *Classes laborieuses et classes dangereuses à Paris pendant la première moitié du XIXe siècle*. Plon, 1958.

Claudel, Camille. *Correspondance*. Edited by Anne Rivière and Bruno Gaudichon. Gallimard, 2014.

Comack, Elizabeth, and Salena Brickey. "Constituting the Violence of Criminalized Women." *Canadian Journal of Criminology and Criminal Justice* 49, no. 1 (2007): 1–36.

Corbin, Alain. *Les filles de noce: Misère sexuelle et prostitution (19e siècle)*. Flammarion, 1982.

Courtwright, David T. *Dark Paradise: A History of Opiate Addiction in America*. Harvard University Press, 2001.

Coutanceau, Roland, and Joanna Smith. *Troubles de la personnalité: Ni psychotiques, ni névrotiques, ni pervers, ni normaux. . . .* Dunod, 2013.

Dijkstra, Bram. *Idols of Perversity: Fantasies of Feminine Evil in Fin-de-Siècle Culture*. Oxford University Press, 1986.

Dodman, Thomas. *What Nostalgia Was: War, Empire, and the Time of a Deadly Emotion*. University of Chicago Press, 2018.

Donovan, James M. *Juries and the Transformation of Criminal Justice in France in the Nineteenth and Twentieth Centuries*. University of North Carolina Press, 2010.

Dormandy, Thomas. *Opium: Reality's Dark Dream*. Yale University Press, 2012.

Dottin-Orsini, Mireille. *Cette femme qu'ils disent fatale: Textes et images de la misogynie fin-de-siècle*. Bernard Grasset, 1993.

Dottin-Orsini, Mireille, and Daniel Grojnowski. *L'imaginaire de la prostitution: De la Bohème à la Belle Époque*. Hermann, 2017.

Downing, Lisa. "Murder in the Feminine: Marie Lafarge and the Sexualization of the Nineteenth-Century Criminal Woman." *Journal of the History of Sexuality* 18, no. 1 (2009): 121–37.

Downing, Lisa. *The Subject of Murder: Gender, Exceptionality and the Modern Killer*. University of Chicago Press, 2013.

Edelman, Nicole. *Voyantes, guérisseuses et visionnaires en France: 1785–1914*. A. Michel, 1997.

Edwards, Rachel, and Keith Reader. *The Papin Sisters*. Oxford University Press, 2001.

Ehrenreich, Barbara, and Deirdre English. *Witches, Midwives and Nurses: A History of Women Healers*. Writers and Readers Publishing Cooperative, 1976.

Eliacheff, Caroline. "Le syndrome de Münchausen par procuration psychique." *Figures de la psychanalyse* 2, no. 12 (2005): 149–64. https://doi.org/10.3917/fp.012.0149.

Ellenberger, Henri F. *The Discovery of the Unconscious: The History and Evolution of Dynamic Psychiatry*. Basic, 1970.

Farge, Arlette, and Thomas Scott-Railton. *The Allure of the Archives*. Yale University Press, 2013.

Ferguson, Eliza Earle. *Gender and Justice: Violence, Intimacy, and Community in Fin-De-Siècle Paris*. Johns Hopkins University Press, 2010.

Finlay, Robert. "The Refashioning of Martin Guerre." *American Historical Review* 93, no. 3 (1988), 553–71.

Finn, Michael. *Figures of the Pre-Freudian Unconscious.* Cambridge University Press, 2017.

Foucault, Michel, ed. *Moi, Pierre Rivière, ayant égorgé ma mère, ma sœur et mon frère: Un cas de parricide au XIXe siècle.* Gallimard/Julliard, 1973.

Freud, Sigmund. *Beyond the Pleasure Principle, Group Psychology and Other Works.* Vol. 18 of *The Standard Edition of the Complete Psychological Works of Sigmund Freud,* edited and translated by J. Strachey et al. Hogarth, 1920–22.

Frydman, Hannah. "Freedom's Sex Problem: Classified Advertising, Law, and the Politics of Reading in Third Republic France." *French Historical Studies* 44, no. 4 (2021): 675–709. https://doi.org/10.1215/00161071-9248720.

Fuchs, Rachel G. *Poor and Pregnant in Paris: Strategies for Survival in the Nineteenth Century.* Rutgers University Press, 1992.

Gelfand, Elissa D. *Imagination in Confinement: Women's Writings from French Prisons.* Cornell University Press, 1983.

Gide, André. *Ne jugez pas.* Gallimard, 1957.

Ginzburg, Carlo. *The Cheese and the Worms: The Cosmos of a Sixteenth-Century Miller.* Translated by John A. Tedeschi and Anne Tedeschi. Penguin, 1992.

Ginzburg, Carlo. "Checking the Evidence: The Judge and the Historian." *Critical Inquiry* 18, no. 1 (1991): 79–92.

Ginzburg, Carlo, and Carlo Poni. "La Micro-Histoire." *Le Débat* 10, no. 17 (1981): 133–36.

Goldstein, Jan. *Console and Classify: The French Psychiatric Profession in the Nineteenth Century.* Cambridge University Press, 1987.

Goldstein, Jan. *Hysteria Complicated by Ecstasy: The Case of Nanette Leroux.* Princeton University Press, 2010.

Gras, Pierre. *Histoire de Dijon.* Privat, 1981.

Guillais, Joëlle. *Crimes of Passion: Dramas of Private Life in Nineteenth-Century France.* Polity, 1990.

Hacking, Ian. *Historical Ontology.* Harvard University Press, 2004.

Hacking, Ian. *Mad Travelers: Reflections on the Reality of Transient Mental Illnesses.* Harvard University Press, 2002.

Harris, Ruth. "Murder Under Hypnosis." *Psychological Medicine* 15, no. 3 (1985): 477–505. doi.org/10.1017/S0033291700031366.

Harris, Ruth. *Murders and Madness: Medicine, Law, and Society in the Fin de Siècle.* Clarendon, 1989.

Harrison, P. J., Philip Cowen, Tom Burns, and Mina Fazel. *Shorter Oxford Textbook of Psychiatry.* 7th ed. Oxford University Press, 2018.

Hartman, Mary S. *Victorian Murderesses: A True History of Thirteen Respectable French and English Women Accused of Unspeakable Crimes.* Robson, 1977.

Hewitt, Jessie. *Institutionalizing Gender: Madness, the Family, and Psychiatric Power in Nineteenth-Century France.* Cornell University Press, 2020.

Homrighaus, Ruth Ellen. "Baby Farming: The Care of Illegitimate Children in England, 1860–1943." PhD diss., University of North Carolina at Chapel Hill, 2003.

Horowitz, Sarah. "Scandalous Friendships: The Dangers of Intimacy in the Stein-
    heil Affair of 1908–1909." *Romanic Review* 110, nos. 1–4 (2019): 247–64.

Illich, Ivan. *Limits to Medicine: Medical Nemesis: The Expropriation of Health.* Boyars,
    1976.

Joseph, Wendy. *Unlawful Killings: Life, Love and Murder: Trials at the Old Bailey.* Dou-
    bleday, 2022.

Kanaan, Richard A., and Simon C. Wessely. "The Origins of Factitious Disorder."
    History of the Human Sciences 23, no. 2 (2010): 68–85.

Kaplan & Sadock's Comprehensive Textbook of Psychiatry. Edited by Benjamin J.
    Sadock, Virginia A. Sadock, and Pedro Ruiz. 10th ed. Wolters Kluwer, 2017.

Krafft-Ebing, Richard von. *Psychopathia Sexualis: The Case Histories.* F. A. Davis,
    1892.

Krakovitch, Odile. *Les femmes bagnardes.* O. Orban, 1990.

Lacapra, Dominic. *History and Criticism.* Cornell University Press, 1985.

Lawrence, Marilyn. "Anorexia Nervosa: The Control Paradox." *Women's Studies
    International Quarterly* 2, no. 1979 (1979): 93–101.

Le Roy Ladurie, Emmanuel. *Montaillou, village occitan de 1294 à 1324.* Gallimard,
    1975.

Le Mée, René. "Une affaire de 'faiseuses d'anges' à la fin du XIXᵉ siècle." *Communi-
    cations: Dénatalité, d'antériorité française, 1880–1914* 44 (1986): 137–74.

Lejeune, Philippe. "Crime et testament: Les autobiographies de criminels au XIXᵉ
    Siècle." *Récits de vie & institutions*, nos. 8–9 (1986): 73–98.

Leys, Ruth. *Trauma: A Genealogy.* University of Chicago Press, 2000.

Lifton, Robert Jay. *The Nazi Doctors: Medical Killing and the Psychology of Genocide.*
    Macmillan, 1986.

Luc, Jean-Noël. *L'invention du jeune enfant au XIXᵉ siècle: De la salle d'asile à l'école
    maternelle.* Belin, 1997.

Marshall, Jonathan W. *Performing Neurology: The Dramaturgy of Dr. Jean-Martin Char-
    cot.* Palgrave Macmillan, 2016.

Martin, Benjamin F. *Crime and Criminal Justice Under the Third Republic: The Shame of
    Marianne.* Louisiana State University Press, 1990.

Maus de Rolley, Thibaut. *Moi, Louis Gaufridy, ayant soufflé plus de mille femmes: Une
    confession de sorcier au XVIIe siècle.* Belles lettres, 2023.

Maza, Sarah C. *Thinking About History.* University of Chicago Press, 2017.

Maza, Sarah C. *Violette Nozière: A Story of Murder in 1930s Paris.* University of Cali-
    fornia Press, 2011.

McCracken, Patti. *The Angel Makers: The True Story of the Most Astonishing Murder
    Ring in History.* Mudlark, 2023.

Meadow, Roy. "Munchausen Syndrome by Proxy: The Hinterland of Child Abuse."
    Lancet 310, no. 8033 (1977): 343–45.

Mermet, Émile. *Annuaire de la presse française.* Chez l'auteur, 1883.

Michel, Louise. *Le Livre du bagne.* Edited by Véronique Fau-Vincenti. Presses univer-
    sitaires de Lyon, 2001.

Millard, Chris. "Concepts, Diagnosis and the History of Medicine: Historicizing
    Ian Hacking and Munchausen Syndrome," *Social History of Medicine* 30, no. 3
    (2017): 567–89.

Motz, Anna. *A Love That Kills: Stories of Forensic Psychology and Female Violence*. Weidenfeld & Nicolson, 2023.

Murat, Laure. *La maison du docteur Blanche: Histoire d'un asile et de ses pensionnaires, de Nerval à Maupassant*. Lattès, 2001.

Murat, Laure. *The Man Who Thought He Was Napoleon: Toward a Political History of Madness*. University of Chicago Press, 2014.

Luc, Jean-Noël. *L'invention du jeune enfant au XIXe siècle: De la salle d'asile à l'école maternelle*. Belin, 1997.

Norris, Anna. *L'écriture du défi: Textes carcéraux féminins du XIXe et du XXe siècles: Entre l'aiguille et la plume*. Summa, 2003.

Nye, Robert A. *Crime, Madness, and Politics in Modern France: The Medical Concept of National Decline*. Princeton University Press, 1984.

Omari, Nejma. "Que toute femme choisisse elle-même sa destinée! Le droit à l'avortement avant la loi Veil." BNF Gallica blog, 15 January 2021. https://gallica.bnf.fr/blog/15012021/que-toute-femme-choisisse-elle-meme-sa-destinee-le-droit-lavortement-avant-la-loi-veil?mode=desktop#block-commentsblock-comment-form-block.

Padwa, Howard. *Social Poison: The Culture and Politics of Opiate Control in Britain and France, 1821–1926*. Johns Hopkins University Press, 2012.

Parssinen, Terry M., and Karren Kerner. "Development of the Disease Model of Drug Addiction in Britain, 1870–1926." *Medical History* 24, no. 3 (1980): 275–96. https://doi.org/10.1017/S0025727300040321.

Perrot, Michelle. "L'affaire Troppmann (1869)." *L'Histoire* 1981, no. 30 (1981): 28–37.

Porret, Michel. *Le sang des lilas: Une mère mélancolique égorge ses quatre enfants en mai 1885 à Genève*. Georg éditeur, 2019.

Praz, Mario. *The Romantic Agony*. Oxford University Press, 1970.

Prendergast, Christopher. "Literature and the City in the Nineteenth Century." In *The Cambridge History of French Literature*, edited by William Burgwinkle, Nicholas Hammond, and Emma Wilson. Cambridge University Press, 2011.

Rabaté, Jean-Michel. "From the History of Perversion to the Trauma of History." In *The Cambridge Introduction to Literature and Psychoanalysis*. Cambridge University Press, 2014.

Repper, Julie. "Munchausen Syndrome by Proxy in Health Care Workers." *Journal of Advanced Nursing* 21, no. 2 (1995): 299–304. https://doi.org/10.1111/J.1365-2648.1995.TB02526.X.

Retaillaud-Bajac, Emmanuelle. *Les paradis perdus: Drogues et usagers de drogues dans la France de l'entre-deux-guerres*. Presses Universitaires de Rennes, 2009.

Richet, Charles. *Traité de Métapsychique*. F. Alcan, 1922.

Roumieux, André. *Artaud et l'asile*. Séguier, 1996.

Salomé, Karine. "Voleur ou assassin? Discours et représentations autour de l'affaire Troppmann (1869–1870)." In *Au Voleur!*, edited by Frédéric Chauvaud and Arnaud-Dominique Houte. Éditions de la Sorbonne, 2014.

Semelaigne, René. *Les Pionniers de la psychiatrie française avant et après Pinel*. J.-B. Baillière et fils, 1930.

Shapiro, Ann-Louise. *Breaking the Codes: Female Criminality in Fin-de-Siècle Paris.* Stanford University Press, 1996.

Sloan Goldberg, Nancy. "The Radicalization of Louise Michel." In *Prison Narratives from Boethius to Zana,* edited by Philip E. Phillips. Palgrave Macmillan, 2014.

Smith, Paul. "Les reconversions des manufactures françaises des tabacs." *Ethnologies* 42, no. 1/2 (2020): 267–95.

Stirling, John, Carole Jenny, Cindy Christian, Roberta A. Hibbard, Nancy D. Kellogg, and Betty S. Spivak. "Beyond Munchausen Syndrome by Proxy: Identification and Treatment of Child Abuse in a Medical Setting." *Pediatrics* 119, no. 5 (2007): 1026–30. https://doi.org/10.1542/PEDS.2007-0563.

Weber, Eugen. *France: Fin de Siècle.* Harvard University Press, 1986.

Wilson, Colette. "City Space and the Politics of Carnival in Zola's *L'Assommoir.*" *French Studies* 58, no. 3 (2004): 343–56.

Wilson, Elizabeth. "The Invisible Flaneur." *New Left Review* 191 (1992): 90–110.

Wilson, Susannah. "To Whom Does a Letter Belong? Psychopathology and Epistolography in the Asylum Letters of Antonin Artaud and Camille Claudel." *Modern Languages Open* 1 (2021): 1–18. https://doi.org/10.3828/mlo.v0i0.360.

Wright, V., É. Anceau, and S. Hazareesingh. *Les Préfets de Gambetta.* Presses de l'université Paris-Sorbonne, 2007.

Yardley, Elizabeth, and David Wilson. "In Search of the 'Angels of Death': Conceptualizing the Contemporary Nurse Healthcare Serial Killer." *Journal of Investigative Psychology and Offender Profiling* 13, no. 1 (2016): 39–55. https://doi.org/10.1002/JIP.1434.

Yvorel, Jean-Jacques. "De la loi 'Lafarge' à la loi de 1916: Aux origines de la pénalisation des stupéfiants." *Psychotropes* 23, no. 2 (2016): 11–23. https://doi.org/10.3917/psyt.222.0009.

Yvorel, Jean-Jacques. "La loi du 12 juillet 1916." *Les cahiers dynamiques* 56, no. 3 (2012): 128–33. https://doi.org/10.3917/lcd.056.0128.

Yvorel, Jean-Jacques. *Les poisons de l'esprit: Drogues et drogués au XIXᵉ siècle.* Quai Voltaire, 1992.

Zemon Davis, Natalie. *The Return of Martin Guerre.* Harvard University Press, 2001.

INDEX